# Depression and Diabetes

*Editors*

**Wayne Katon**
*Department of Psychiatry and Behavioral Sciences, University
of Washington School of Medicine, Seattle, WA, USA*

**Mario Maj**
*Department of Psychiatry, University of Naples SUN,
Naples, Italy*

**Norman Sartorius**
*Association for the Improvement of Mental Health
Programmes, Geneva, Switzerland*

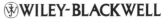
A John Wiley & Sons, Ltd., Publication

This edition first published 2010 © 2010, John Wiley & Sons, Ltd.

Wiley-Blackwell is an imprint of John Wiley & Sons, formed by the merger of Wiley's global Scientific, Technical and Medical business with Blackwell Publishing.

*Registered office:* John Wiley & Sons Ltd, The Atrium, Southern Gate, Chichester, West Sussex, PO19 8SQ, UK

*Other Editorial Offices:*
9600 Garsington Road, Oxford, OX4 2DQ, UK
111 River Street, Hoboken, NJ 07030-5774, USA

For details of our global editorial offices, for customer services and for information about how to apply for permission to reuse the copyright material in this book please see our website at www.wiley.com/wiley-blackwell

*Library of Congress Cataloguing-in-Publication Data*

Depression and diabetes / editors, Wayne Katon, Mario Maj, Norman Sartorius.
    p. ; cm.
    Includes bibliographical references and index.
    Summary: "Depression and Diabetes is the first book devoted to the interaction between these common disorders. World leaders in diabetes, depression, and public health synthesize current evidence, including some previously unpublished data, in a concise, easy-to-read format. They provide an overview of the epidemiology, pathogenesis, medical costs, management, and public health and cultural implications of the comorbidity between depression and diabetes. The book describes how the negative consequences of depression in diabetes could be avoided, given that effective depression treatments for diabetic patients are available."–Provided by publisher.
    ISBN 978-0-470-68838-0 (paper)
    1. Diabetes–Treatment. 2. Diabetes–Psychological aspects. 3. Depression, Mental–Treatment. I. Katon, Wayne. II. Maj, Mario, 1953- III. Sartorius, N.
    [DNLM: 1. Depressive Disorder. 2. Diabetes Complications. WM 171 D42238 2010]
    RC660.D43 2010
    616.4'6206–dc22

                                2010016178

ISBN: 9780470688380

A catalogue record for this book is available from the British Library.

Set in 10/12 Pt Times by Thomson Digital, Noida, India.
Printed and bound in Singapore by Fabulous Printers Pte Ltd.

Second Impression   2011

# Depression and Diabetes

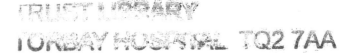

## World Psychiatric Association titles on Depression

In recent years, there has been a growing awareness of the multiple interrelationships between depression and various physical diseases. This series of volumes dealing with the comorbidity of depression with diabetes, heart disease and cancer provides an update of currently available evidence on these interrelationships.

**Depression and Diabetes**
*Edited by Wayne Katon, Mario Maj and Norman Sartorius*
ISBN: 9780470688380

**Depression and Heart Disease**
*Edited by Alexander Glassman, Mario Maj and Norman Sartorius*
ISBN: 9780470710579

**Depression and Cancer**
*Edited by David W. Kissane, Mario Maj and Norman Sartorius*
ISBN: 9780470689660

Related WPA title on depression:

**Depressive Disorders, 3e**
*Edited by Helen Herrman, Mario Maj and Norman Sartorius*
ISBN: 9780470987209

For all other WPA titles published by John Wiley & Sons Ltd, please visit the following website pages:

http://eu.wiley.com/WileyCDA/Section/id-305609.html

http://eu.wiley.com/WileyCDA/Section/id-303180.html

# Contents

# List of Contributors

**Juliana Chan**   Hong Kong Institute of Diabetes and Obesity; Department of Medicine and Therapeutics, Chinese University of Hong Kong, Prince of Wales Hospital, Hong Kong SAR, China

**Paul Ciechanowski**   Department of Psychiatric and Behavioral Sciences, University of Washington School of Medicine, Seattle, WA, USA

**Leonard E. Egede**   Department of Medicine, Center for Health Disparities Research, Medical University of South Carolina; and Center for Disease Prevention and Health Interventions for Diverse Populations, Ralph H. Johnson VA Medical Center, Charleston, SC, USA

**Christina van der Feltz-Cornelis**   Department of Clinical and Developmental Psychology, University of Tilburg; Centre of Top Clinical Care for Somatoform Disorder, GGZ Breburg, Breda; Trimbos Institute, Utrecht, The Netherlands

**Richard Hellman**   Department of Medicine, University of Missouri, Kansas City, MO, USA

**Norbert Hermanns**   Research Institute, Mergentheim, Germany

**Khalida Ismail**   Department of Psychological Medicine, Institute of Psychiatry, King's College London, London, UK

**Wayne Katon**   Department of Psychiatry and Behavioral Sciences, University of Washington School of Medicine, Seattle, WA, USA

**Cathy E. Lloyd**   Faculty of Health and Social Care, The Open University, Milton Keynes, UK

**Hairong Nan**   Hong Kong Institute of Diabetes and Obesity, Chinese University of Hong Kong, Prince of Wales Hospital, Hong Kong SAR, China

**Arie Nouwen**   School of Psychology, University of Birmingham, Birmingham, UK

**Frans Pouwer**   Centre for Research on Psychology in Somatic Diseases (CoRPS), Tilburg University, Tilburg, The Netherlands

**Rose Ting**   Department of Medicine and Therapeutics, Chinese University of Hong Kong, Prince of Wales Hospital, Hong Kong SAR, China

**Leigh Underwood**   Greater Western Area Health Service/Centre for Rural and Remote Mental Health, New South Wales, Australia

**Kirsty Winkley**   Diabetes and Mental Health Unit, King's College London, and Institute of Psychiatry, London, UK

# Preface

The association between depression and diabetes was first described in the seventeenth century by Thomas Willis, an English physician and anatomist, who stated, 'Diabetes is caused by sadness or long sorrow'. Indeed, in modern times, a systematic review found that depression earlier in life increased the risk of development of type 2 diabetes by up to 37%.

Evidence of a bidirectional relationship between depression and diabetes has also been recently documented in large prospective studies. Comorbid depression is associated with an increased risk of poor glycemic control, diabetes complications and mortality. Incident diabetes complications have also been found to be risk factors for subsequent development of depressive episodes.

In this book, authors on the cutting edge of research in patients with comorbid depression and diabetes describe the most up-to-date findings. The importance of the research on depression and diabetes has been emphasized in recent years because of the modern-day epidemic of obesity and diabetes that is emerging in both high and low income countries. The direct medical and indirect personal and familial costs of this epidemic are starting to get international attention. In the United States, the cost of diabetes already is estimated to represent about 10% of all medical costs and is expected to increase by 50–100% over the next decade. The public health importance and the scientific issues related to the comorbidity of depression and diabetes have led to an international scientific collaboration, the Diabetes and Depression Initiative, which is bringing together a number of organizations and experts, several of whom have participated in the production of this volume.

In this exciting new text, Cathy Lloyd and colleagues describe the epidemiology of depression and diabetes, including the prevalence and course of depression in patients with type 1 and 2 diabetes, evidence of bidirectional links between these two disorders, and associations of depression with adverse health habits (i.e. smoking and obesity), poor disease control, medical complications and mortality. Khalida Ismail reviews the putative biologic links between depression and diabetes, which may explain why depression in early life is a risk factor for development of type 2 diabetes as well as an important factor in risk of complications and mortality in those with type 2 diabetes.

Leonard Egede reviews the extensive data on the increased medical and personal, familial and employment-related costs of comorbid depression and diabetes. These data are extremely important to health policy planners in emphasizing the potential benefit of screening patients with diabetes for depression. The epidemiologic data have shown that depression is a risk factor for poor disease control, diabetes macrovascular and microvascular complications and mortality, and Egede's data add to these findings by showing the high direct medical and indirect costs, such as days off work and decreased productivity.

Wayne Katon and Christina van der Felz-Cornelis describe the clinical trials that have been completed in patients with depression and diabetes, including pharmacologic, psychotherapy and collaborative care trials. This extensive research demonstrates that depression can be effectively treated by both evidence-based depression-focused psychotherapy and antidepressant medications, and that collaborative care is an effective health service model to deliver these treatments to large, primary care-based populations. Collaborative care is associated not only with improved quality of depression care and depressive outcomes, but also with a high likelihood of savings in total medical costs.

Richard Hellman and Paul Ciechanowski review the important patient–physician factors that need to be emphasized to provide guideline-level diabetes care. Their chapter focuses on the interaction of depression, cognitive dysfunction, glycemic control and diabetes complications and provides state-of-the-art recommendations about how to improve quality of biopsychosocial care for patients with diabetes.

In the final chapter, Juliana Chan and colleagues describe the important cultural issues in patients with depression and diabetes in both high and low income countries. Public health campaigns aimed at decreasing the incidence of obesity and type 2 diabetes and improving screening and treatment of depression will clearly need to understand the sociocultural causes and meanings of these illnesses in diverse populations.

This volume is part of a WPA series focusing on the comorbidity of depression with various physical diseases. Forthcoming volumes will deal with depression and heart disease and depression and cancer.

**Wayne Katon**
**Mario Maj**
**Norman Sartorius**

# CHAPTER 1

# The Epidemiology of Depression and Diabetes

## Cathy E. Lloyd
*Faculty of Health and Social Care, The Open University, Milton Keynes, UK*

## Norbert Hermanns
*Research Institute, Mergentheim, Germany*

## Arie Nouwen
*School of Psychology, University of Birmingham, Birmingham, UK*

## Frans Pouwer
*Centre for Research on Psychology in Somatic Diseases (CoRPS), Tilburg University, Tilburg, The Netherlands*

## Leigh Underwood
*Greater Western Area Health Service/Centre for Rural and Remote Mental Health, New South Wales, Australia*

## Kirsty Winkley
*Diabetes and Mental Health Unit, King's College London, and Institute of Psychiatry, London, UK*

In recent years there has been a heightened interest in the psychological well-being of people with diabetes. Current epidemiological evidence suggests that at least one third of them suffer from clinically relevant depressive disorders [1–3]. Furthermore, people with depressive disorders have an increased risk of developing diabetes [4].

*Depression and Diabetes*   Edited by Wayne Katon, Mario Maj and Norman Sartorius
© 2010 John Wiley & Sons, Ltd

Indeed, the prognosis of both diabetes and depression – in terms of severity of disease, complications, treatment resistance and mortality – as well as the costs to both the individual and society [5] is worse for either disease when they are comorbid than it is when they occur separately [6, 7]. However, in spite of the huge impact of comorbid depression and diabetes on the individual and its importance as a public health problem, questions still remain as to the nature of the relationship, its causes and consequences, as well as potential ways of preventing and treating these two conditions. This chapter aims to outline the epidemiological evidence as it stands, as well as point the way for future research in this area.

## RATES OF DEPRESSION IN PEOPLE WITH DIABETES

Depression is usually defined by the number of symptoms present, usually within the past two weeks. In order to diagnose major depression using DSM-IV or ICD-10 criteria, a clinical interview is conducted and a number of symptoms have to be present (Table 1.1). Most epidemiological research on the prevalence of depression uses self-report instruments (for example the Centre for Epidemiologic Studies – Depression Scale [8] or the recently devised Patient Health Questionnaire – 9, PHQ-9 [9]) for detecting depression or depressive symptomatology, and most instruments that are used measure symptoms that approximate clinical levels of disorder (Table 1.1).

Rates of depression in people with diabetes are significantly increased and are thought to be at least doubled for those with diabetes compared to those without any chronic disease [1]. A recent report from the World Health Survey [10] estimated the prevalence of depression (based on ICD-10 criteria) in 245, 404 individuals from 60 countries around the world. The overall one-year prevalence of self-reported symptoms of depression in individuals with diabetes was 9.3%. This study showed that the greatest decrements in self-reported health were observed in those with both depression and diabetes, more so than those with depression and any other chronic disease [10] (Figure 1.1).

Other studies have reported prevalence rates of depression of 24–30% [1, 2, 11]. Recently it has been suggested that although up to

**Table 1.1**  Symptoms listed in the DSM-IV criteria for major depressive disorder and symptoms of depression measured using self-report instruments

**DSM-IV criteria (at least five symptoms present nearly every day for 2 wk and causing significant distress or functional impairment)**

Depressed mood
Markedly diminished interest or pleasure in all or almost all activities
Significant weight loss/gain or decreased/increased appetite
Insomnia or hypersomnia
Psychomotor agitation or retardation
Fatigue or loss of energy
Feelings of worthlessness/guilt
Diminished ability to concentrate/make decisions
Recurrent thoughts of death or suicide

**Symptoms of depression measured using self-report instruments**

Feeling sad/depressed mood
Inability to sleep
Early waking
Lack of interest/enjoyment
Tiredness/lack of energy
Loss of appetite
Feelings of guilt/worthlessness
Recurrent thoughts about death/suicide

DSM-IV criteria extracted from the *Diagnostic and Statistical Manual of Mental Disorders,* Fourth Edition, Text Revision, Copyright 2000. American Psychiatric Association.

30% of individuals with diabetes report depressive symptoms, only about 10% have major depression [12]. However, the published studies differ widely in terms of the methods used to measure depression, which makes any conclusions premature. Rates of depressive symptoms have been found to be higher in those studies where self-report instruments were used compared to diagnostic interviews [1]. Furthermore, in a recent report, Gendelman *et al.* [13] showed that prevalence rates were even higher if reports of elevated symptoms were combined with the use of antidepressant medication. This suggests that the available evidence should be considered with particular methodological differences in case ascertainment kept in mind.

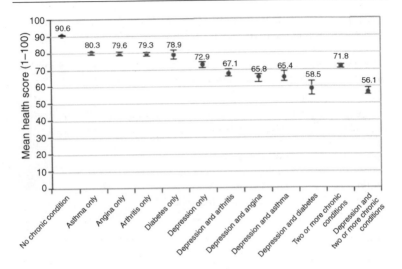

**Figure 1.1** Global mean health by disease status. (Saba Moussavi et al., Depression, chronic diseases and decrements in health: results from the World Health Surveys, The Lancet, 2007, by permission of Elsevier)

Rates of depression have been found to be particularly high in individuals with type 2 diabetes, with less evidence to suggest that rates are also increased in those with type 1 diabetes [3]. Any potential differences are confounded by age, and it is known that older age is a risk factor for higher prevalence of depression in those with other health problems [14, 15]. There may also be an increased prevalence of psychological morbidity in young adults with type 1 diabetes [16–19]. Some reports have indicated that the prevalence of depression does not appear to differ according to type of diabetes [1, 20, 21]. One study [22] reported that those with major depression were more likely to be on insulin treatment rather than on oral agents or diet alone, and this may be related to the increased burden of the self-management regimen in these individuals.

## INTERNATIONAL VARIATIONS IN RATES OF DEPRESSION IN PEOPLE WITH DIABETES

There may be regional/cultural differences in the prevalence of depression. However, this is difficult to establish with available data. Much of the research to date has been on the comparison of prevalence rates generally, and few published studies address culture or ethnicity as a specific factor within or across populations. Of those reports, studies have suggested that individuals from African American backgrounds have higher rates of diabetes and depression compared with Caucasian populations [23, 24]. Other studies have shown that Hispanic people have higher levels of comorbid depression compared with African Americans or Caucasian individuals [25–28]. Several studies have suggested that comorbid depression may also be much more common in native Americans with type 2 diabetes [29, 30].

In one of the few published studies of comorbid depression in the developing world, carried out in Bangladesh, Asghar *et al.* [29] reported that nearly one third (29% males, 30% females) of those with diabetes had clinically significant levels of depression, compared with only 6% of males and 15% of females without diabetes. In Pakistan, levels of depression have been reported to be lower, with prevalence rates of nearly 15% amongst those with diabetes compared to 5% amongst those without diabetes [31]. Prevalence rates in Europe have been shown to vary, although consistently higher in people with diabetes compared to those without [32, 33]. High rates of depression have also been observed in Australia in both individuals with type 1 and type 2 diabetes [11, 34].

It is clear that, although there may well be international variations in rates of comorbid depression and diabetes, there remains further work to be done to clarify whether those variations reflect socioeconomic/ other environmental differences, whether race or culture play a part, or whether at least some of this difference is related to variations in assessment methods or the cultural applicability of those measurement tools. These possibilities still need to be fully examined in future studies.

## RISK FACTORS FOR DEPRESSION IN PEOPLE WITH DIABETES

A range of factors may be implicated in increasing the risk of developing depressive symptoms, both in terms of an initial episode of depression and with regard to the persistence, recurrence and severity of depressive episodes. A number of risk factors identified in individuals without diabetes also apply to those with diabetes, although others may differ. Some of the key risk factors that have been identified are listed in Table 1.2. Elevated depression levels have been found in general populations in women, younger people and also those of older age (especially those with physical health problems), individuals living alone, those who report a lack of social support, and those who have lower socioeconomic status. In individuals with diabetes, the following additional risk factors for depression have been found to be important: occurrence of late or acute complications, persistently poor glycaemic control and insulin therapy in type 2 diabetes [35, 36] (Table 1.2).

In the general population, risk factors for an *initial* depressive episode include gender [37], major stressful life events [38–40] and socioeconomic conditions [41]. Maternal depression has been shown to increase the risk for depression in children and adolescents [42, 43], although this has not been confirmed in other studies [16]. Low birth weight and foetal undernutrition have also been associated with both depression and diabetes [44, 45]. Other factors, including lifestyle and health behaviours, may also play a part in increasing risk for depression in people with diabetes. However, the temporal association between these variables remains unclear and requires further investigation.

**Table 1.2**   Risk factors for depression in diabetes

| Non-diabetes specific risk factors | Diabetes specific risk factors |
| --- | --- |
| Female gender | Manifestation of diabetes |
| Lack of social support | Occurrence of late complications |
| Low socioeconomic status | Persistent poor glycaemic control |
| Younger age; older age and physical health problems | Need for insulin therapy in type 2 diabetes |
| Occurrence of critical life events | Hypoglycaemia problems |

A number of studies have reported a greater prevalence of depression in women with both type 1 diabetes and type 2 diabetes, similar to that observed in the general population [16, 21, 46]. A recent study showed even greater differences between men and women when use of antidepressant medication was included [13]. Indeed, medication use was almost twice as common in women with type 1 diabetes compared to men. There may be gender differences in the experience of depressive symptoms as well as in the reporting of symptoms and help-seeking behaviour. However, there are few studies that have examined these issues in depth [20, 47].

Although depression is not a part of normal ageing [48, 49], prevalence rates of severe depressive episodes/major depressive disorder are higher amongst certain groups of older people, in particular, individuals with a comorbid medical illness [50]. However, to date, little epidemiological data has been available with which to examine rates of depression in older people with diabetes [14, 15, 33, 51]. To further complicate the picture, several studies have reported that depressive symptoms are more common in younger individuals, in both type 1 and type 2 diabetes [16, 52]. Collins et al. [51] also reported lower rates of depression in older individuals with type 1 diabetes, suggesting that age might have a protective effect.

Recurrence of depression is common in people with diabetes, and episodes are likely to last longer [46, 53, 54]. In one five-year follow-up study, Lustman et al. [55] found that recurrence or persistence of major depression occurred in 23 (92%) participants, with an average of 4.8 episodes, after an eight-week treatment with nortriptyline. Kovacs et al. [53] found that episodes of major depressive disorder lasted longer in adolescents with type 1 diabetes than in control participants, although rates of recovery were similar.

The specific factors associated with recurrence of depression remain unclear. Gender has not been found to be associated with the number of episodes or the severity of recurrence or chronicity of depression [56], and the association between stress and depressive episodes appears to be less pronounced over time [57–60]. The evidence would suggest that stress is either no longer important in the triggering of subsequent depressive episodes or that weaker, and therefore more frequent, stressors would suffice [61]. If confirmed, this would mean that the relatively minor stresses of living with diabetes may be enough to trigger a depressive episode in people vulnerable to depression. To date, both general stressors [27] and diabetes-related emotional problems and distress have been linked with higher levels of depressive symptoms [27, 32].

Diabetes-specific risk factors for depression include comorbidity of diabetes-related complications, in particular vascular complications [62–64]. Knowledge of having type 2 diabetes [65–67], longer duration of diabetes [68, 69], more demanding regimens, low levels of daily activities [70–72], higher dependency [73], nutrition (e.g. low intake of omega-3 fatty acids) [74], smoking [75], obesity [76] and perceived burden of diabetes [77, 78] have all been postulated as risk factors, but the epidemiological evidence remains limited. Potential risk factors for depression in people with diabetes often interact with each other and with other factors. For example, the relationship between duration of diabetes and depression may be confounded by the number of complications present.

A small number of studies has examined whether the presence of diabetes *per se* increases the risk of depression in people with type 2 diabetes [14, 33, 79–84]. A recent meta-analysis, which included these studies [85], demonstrated there was only a modest (15%) increased risk of developing depression in people with diabetes. However, this meta-analysis only contained seven studies and no distinction was made whether a diagnosis of depression was used or questionnaires. When examining studies where a diagnosis of depression was made separately from studies where self-reported symptoms were used, the risk of developing depression was 48% and only 20% in the questionnaire studies. Clearly the temporal association between diabetes and depression warrants further attention in long-term prospective studies.

## DEPRESSION AS A RISK FACTOR FOR DIABETES

Mezuk *et al.* [85] reported data showing that depression may be an important risk factor for developing type 2 diabetes. Depression was associated with a 60% increased risk of developing type 2 diabetes.

The link between depression and diabetes was made as early as the seventeenth century, when the famous English physician T. Willis (1621–1675) noted that diabetes often appeared among patients who had experienced significant life stresses, sadness or long sorrow [86]. Whether depression increases the risk of type 1 diabetes is currently unknown. However, recent studies have suggested that people with depression are more vulnerable to the development of type 2 diabetes [85, 87], thereby confirming Willis' hypothesis.

It is important to recognize that depression is not only associated with an increased risk for the development of type 2 diabetes, but is also an established risk factor for cardiovascular disease [88, 89] and several features of the metabolic syndrome, particularly hypertension, abdominal obesity and low HDL cholesterol [90, 91]. Several hypotheses have been put forward regarding the pathophysiological mechanisms that could explain the increased risk of type 2 diabetes in depressed subjects. For example, increased activity of the hypothalamic-pituitary-adrenal (HPA) axis and sympathetic nervous system might play a role; these are examined elsewhere in this volume.

Depression may also increase the risk for type 2 diabetes via behavioural mechanisms. It is well known that the most important risk factor for type 2 diabetes is obesity [92], and that physical inactivity further increases this risk [93]. Interestingly, data from the Heart and Soul Study [89] showed that the association between depression and incident cardiovascular events was largely explained by behavioural factors, particularly physical inactivity.

In summary, the evidence to date suggests that depression may indeed increase the risk of developing type 2 diabetes. However, the mechanisms via which this may occur still require investigation. The link between depression and the development of type 1 diabetes remains unclear.

## DEPRESSIVE SYMPTOMATOLOGY AND GLYCAEMIC CONTROL

People with diabetes are expected to carry out lifelong multiple self-care tasks (including self-monitoring of blood glucose, dietary modifications, exercising and managing medications) in order to achieve optimal glycaemic control and so reduce the risk of developing serious complications. Intensive insulin and medication regimes and structured education programmes are effective in improving glycaemic control, decreasing cardiovascular risk and reducing diabetes complications in both type 1 and type 2 diabetes [94, 95]. However, for some individuals there are likely to be both psychological and social barriers to maintaining good glycaemic control over time.

Depression is associated with adverse outcomes in diabetes, and there is some evidence to suggest that depression worsens glycaemic control because it worsens self-care [96, 97]. For example, in one prospective study of approximately 4000 people with diabetes, depression was associated with poor concordance with oral medication taking, even in those with reasonable glycaemic control levels prior to the study [98]. Numerous studies, usually cross-sectional, suggest depression is associated with suboptimal glycaemic control, although in a systematic review the effect size was moderate [99]. Of the few prospective studies [100–103], only one [103] demonstrated a clear association between depression at baseline and persistently higher HbA1c levels over a four-year period. However, this study had some limitations, as it did not consider potential mediating factors, such as medication taking and diabetes self-management.

So far, the exact mechanism linking depression, glycaemic control, morbidity and mortality has not been established. The 'depression leading to poor self-care' hypothesis does not seem to tell the whole story. For example, when depression is treated in diabetes, whether by pharmacotherapy or using psychological techniques, depression is improved, but not necessarily glycaemic control [46, 104–110]. This suggests that depression could influence morbidity and mortality via other pathways, such as those involved in cardiovascular disease and lipid dysregulation. Future prospective studies measuring a range of biopsychosocial factors will allow us to unpick these complex interactions.

## MILD DEPRESSION AND OTHER PSYCHOLOGICAL COMORBIDITIES IN PEOPLE WITH DIABETES

Having mild or subthreshold depression may have a disproportionate impact on people with diabetes. Owing to the effects on diabetes self-management, what may be regarded as 'subclinical' in someone without diabetes may be seen as of great clinical importance when combined with diabetes [5]. This 'mild' depression may not just be the result of living with diabetes, but also a response to stresses and life events independent of diabetes (e.g. marital problems, work-related stresses) that may interact with diabetes.

Depressive symptoms commonly occur in other psychiatric disorders, such as eating and anxiety disorders. Depressive symptoms are common to young women with eating disorders: they are not separately diagnosed, but regarded as part of the illness/diagnosis, and affect approximately 30–50% of people with anorexia nervosa and 50% of those with bulimia nervosa [111]. Eating disorders associated with poor diabetes self-care, such as underdosing or omission of insulin to promote weight loss, occur disproportionately in pre-teen girls with diabetes [112–115].

Anxiety is common in diabetes populations and is frequently associated with depression [7, 20, 51, 52]. A recent systematic review found that around 14% of people with diabetes have generalized anxiety disorder, but subclinical anxiety and symptoms were more common and affected 27% and 40% respectively [116]. The presence of comorbid depression or anxiety has been associated with increased somatic symptoms of disease, which has important implications for treatment [7]. Diabetes-specific psychological problems, such as fear of self-injecting insulin or self-testing blood glucose (which may or may not be full-blown needle phobia) and fear of complications, are all associated with anxiety and depression [117–119]. Fears regarding hypoglycaemia and psychological insulin resistance are also common, but their relationship with depression is less clear [120, 121].

Several recent reports have indicated that psychosocial factors, including emotional problems related to diabetes, are associated with elevated levels of depression [32, 122]. These studies have used the Problem Areas in Diabetes (PAID) scale, which was developed to measure diabetes-related emotional distress, often referred to as 'diabetes burn-out', in individuals with either type 1 or type 2 diabetes [77]. Research has shown strong correlations between depressive symptomatology and diabetes-related distress. However, whilst many of those with high depression symptoms also report high

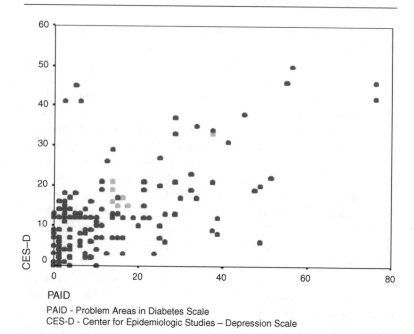

**Figure 1.2** The overlap between symptoms of depression and diabetes-related distress. (With permission from Skinner TC, Combined Universities Centre for Rural Health, Australia)

diabetes-related emotional distress, there are also a significant number of individuals who only have either one or the other (Figure 1.2). Further studies are required in order to tease out the relative importance of different psychological morbidity and the impact on diabetes care.

## LONGER-TERM OUTCOMES AND THE IMPACT OF DEPRESSION IN DIABETES

Depression in diabetes is associated with greater morbidity and mortality and poorer quality of life. Evidence shows that depressive symptoms are associated with less dietary self-care, poorer physical and mental functioning, increased use of health services and, in type 2 diabetes, poorer concordance with oral medication recommendations [96, 123].

As diabetes affects the economically active, there is the potential for loss of economic or social roles, affecting marital and family life, causing isolation and stigmatization, which may also engender depression. People who are depressed often have negative views regarding their diabetes, and these may perpetuate adverse coping behaviours and increase the likelihood of poor outcomes [124–126].

Depressive symptoms are more common in people with diabetes complications, although the causal direction of this relationship is unclear [33, 64]. Studies from an onset cohort of type 1 diabetes have demonstrated a prospective association between prior depressive symptoms and the onset of coronary artery disease [127, 128]. A similar association between depression and onset of retinopathy has also been identified in a study of children with diabetes [129]. Although depression is a risk factor for the onset of type 2 diabetes [87] and cardiovascular disease [130], people who experience diabetes complications suffer a loss of function that might lead to depression.

The wider literature supports a bidirectional relationship between depression and vascular disease [131]. Macro- and micro-vascular problems typically co-occur in diabetes, such as erectile dysfunction and diabetic foot disease, but it can be difficult to detect early signs of micro-vascular damage, so establishing the relationship between depression and the onset of conditions such as neuropathy is problematic.

There have been numerous prospective studies demonstrating an association between depression and mortality in people with (predominantly type 2) diabetes, which suggests a synergistic interactive effect of depression on cardiovascular mortality [100, 101, 132]. In a study in the United Kingdom, major and minor depressive episodes increased mortality risk threefold in a cohort of people with diabetes and their first foot ulcer at 18 months [101]. In the United States, the Pathways Study demonstrated a 1.67 and 2.30-fold increase in mortality at three years in those with minor and major depression, respectively [100]. Another study reported a 50% increased risk of death among people with diabetes, but no increased risk of death from cardiovascular disease [133].

The Hispanic Established Population for the Epidemiologic Study of the Elderly (EPESE) reported that depressed individuals were almost five times more likely to die and were significantly more likely to develop early onset of diabetes complications at seven years follow-up [134]. Finally, the US National Health and Nutrition Examination Survey (NHANES) compared people with diabetes and depression to people with diabetes and no depression and other non-diabetes groups at eight years follow-up, and determined a 2.50-fold increase in all-cause mortality in the depressed diabetes group and a 2.43-fold increase in coronary heart disease mortality [5].

In another study using the NHANES data (Figures 1.3 and 1.4), Zhang *et al.* [132] also demonstrated a strong association between depressive symptoms and increased mortality in people with diabetes, which they did not observe in those without diabetes, even after adjusting for sociodemographic and lifestyle factors. These findings have important implications for the care of people with comorbid depression and diabetes.

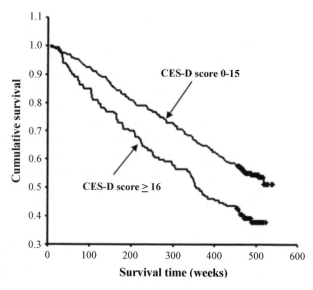

**Figure 1.3**   Survival functions in a diabetic population stratified by Center for Epidemiologic Studies-Depression (CES-D) Scale score. (Xuanping Zhang *et al.*, Depressive symptoms and mortality among persons with and without diabetes, American Journal of Epidemiology, 2005, by permission of Oxford University Press)

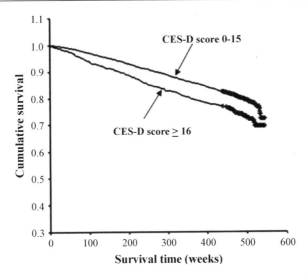

**Figure 1.4**  Survival functions in a non-diabetic population stratified by Centers for Epidemiologic Studies-Depression (CES-D) Scale score. (Xuanping Zhang *et al.*, Depressive symptoms and mortality among persons with and without diabetes, American Journal of Epidemiology, 2005, by permission of Oxford University Press)

## CONCLUSIONS

Current epidemiological evidence demonstrates that people with diabetes have an increased risk of experiencing one or more depressive episodes in their lifetime and that this can have serious adverse consequences. This increased prevalence may be related to people with diabetes experiencing longer lasting or more recurrent depressive episodes, rather than an increased risk of developing depression *per se*.

A range of potential risk factors for this increased vulnerability has been postulated. However, much of the evidence cited is from cross-sectional studies and so the temporal relationship between the two conditions is yet to be fully determined. In particular, the role of a previous history of depression in future episodes remains unclear, and large population-based prospective studies are needed to examine this further.

The methods used to assess depressive symptoms have varied between studies and it is not clear whether different conclusions would be reached if more stringent diagnostic criteria were used. Given the known inter- and intra-national differences in prevalence rates, further research needs to be conducted in order to tease out whether these variations are due to the cultural inapplicability of particular measurement tools, or whether there are 'true' differences related to wider socioeconomic factors and/or cultural/ethnic marginalization.

People from ethnic minorities, lower socioeconomic status, or those who are obese also tend to have more mental health problems [135–137]. However, it is not clear how these factors exert their influence on diabetes outcomes, and this is an area where there has been little research.

Outcomes for people with depression and diabetes are frequently poor, and this includes the impact on self-management, glycaemic control and other comorbidities, including diabetes complications. However, the mechanisms mediating the associations between these and psychological and social factors remain poorly understood and require further investigation.

There is likely to be a complex biopsychosocial explanation. However, prospective evidence is not yet available. Further studies are required in order to tease out the relative importance of different psychological morbidities and their impact on glycaemic control, the development of diabetes complications, mortality and the management of diabetes.

## ACKNOWLEDGEMENTS

The authors would like to thank the following individuals for their thoughtful and constructive comments on this chapter: Kate Gilbert, Founder of the Type 1 Diabetes Network, Australia; Christos Lionis, University of Crete, Greece; Robert Peveler, University of Southampton, UK: Timothy Skinner, Combined Universities Centre for Rural Health, Australia; Corinne Stoop, Trimbos Institute, The Netherlands; and Dorothy Thomas, Royal Flying Doctor Service of Australia.

# REFERENCES

1. Anderson, R.J., Freedland, K.E., Clouse, R.E., and Lustman, P.J. (2001) The prevalence of co-morbid depression in adults with diabetes. *Diabetes Care*, **6**, 1069–1078.
2. Ali, S., Stone, M., Peters, J. *et al.* (2006) The prevalence of co-morbid depression in adults with Type 2 diabetes: a systematic review and meta-analysis. *Diabet. Med.*, **23**, 1165–1173.
3. Barnard, K., Skinner, T., and Peveler, R. (2006) The prevalence of co-morbid depression in adults with Type 1 diabetes: systematic literature review. *Diabet. Med.*, **23**, 445–448.
4. Pouwer, F., Beekman, T.F., Nijpels, G. *et al.* (2003) Rates and risks for co-morbid depression in patients with Type 2 diabetes mellitus: results from a community-based study. *Diabetologia*, **46**, 892–898.
5. Simon, G., Katon, W., Lin, E. *et al.* (2005) Diabetes complications and depression as predictors of health service costs. *Gen. Hosp. Psychiatry*, **27**, 344–351.
6. Egede, L.E., Nietert, P.J., and Zheng, D. (2005) Depression and all-cause and coronary mortality among adults with and without diabetes. *Diabetes Care*, **28**, 1339–1345.
7. Katon, W., Lin, E.H., and Kroenke, K. (2007) The association of depression and anxiety with medical symptom burden in patients with chronic medical illness. *Gen. Hosp. Psychiatry*, **29**, 147–155.
8. Radloff, L.S. (1977) A self-report depression scale for research in the general population. *Appl. Psych. Meas.*, **1**, 385–401.
9. Kroenke, K., Spitzer, R.L., and Williams, J.B. (2001) The PHQ-9: validity of a brief depression severity measure. *J. Gen. Intern. Med.*, **16**, 606–613.
10. Moussavi, S., Chatterji, S., Verdes, E. *et al.* (2007) Depression, chronic diseases, and decrements in health: results from the World Health Surveys. *Lancet*, **370**, 851–858.
11. Goldney, R., Phillips, P., Gisher, L., and Wilson, D. (2004) Diabetes, depression and quality of life. *Diabetes Care*, **27**, 1066–1070.
12. Egede, L. (2004) Diabetes, major depression, and functional disability among U.S. adults. *Diabetes Care*, **27**, 421–428.
13. Gendelman, N., Snell-Bergeon, J.K., McFann, K. *et al.* (2009) Prevalence and correlates of depression in individuals with and without Type 1 diabetes. *Diabetes Care*, **32**, 575–579.
14. Maraldi, C., Volpato, S., Penninx, B. *et al.* (2007) Diabetes mellitus, glycemic control, and incident depressive symptoms among 70- to

79-year-old persons: the health, aging, and body composition study. *Arch. Gen. Med.*, **167**, 1137–1144.

15. Nouwen, A. and Oyebode, J.R. (2009) Depression and diabetes in older adults, in *Diabetes in Old Age* (ed. A. Sinclair), John Wiley & Sons Ltd, Chichester, pp. 385–401.

16. Kovacs, M., Goldston, D., Obrosky, D.S., and Bonar, L.K. (1997) Psychiatric disorders in youths with IDDM: rates and risk factors. *Diabetes Care*, **20**, 36–44.

17. Bryden, K.S., Neil, A., Mayou, R.A. *et al.* (1999) Eating habits, body weight, and insulin misuse. *Diabetes Care*, **22**, 1956–1960.

18. Northam, E.A., Matthews, L.K., Anderson, P.J. *et al.* (2004) Psychiatric morbidity and health outcome in Type 1 diabetes – perspectives from a prospective longitudinal study. *Diabet. Med.*, **22**, 152–157.

19. Lawrence, J.M., Standiford, D.A., Loots, B. *et al.* (2006) Prevalence and correlates of depressed mood among youth with diabetes: the SEARCH for diabetes in youth study. *J. Pediatrics*, **117**, 1348–1358.

20. Lloyd, C.E., Dyer, P.H., and Barnett, A.H. (2000) Prevalence of symptoms of depression and anxiety in a diabetes clinic population. *Diabet. Med.*, **17**, 198–202.

21. Engum, A., Mykletun, A., Midthjell, K. *et al.* (2005) Depression and diabetes: a large population-based study of sociodemographic, lifestyle, and clinical factors associated with depression in type 1 and type 2 diabetes. *Diabetes Care*, **28**, 1904–1909.

22. Katon, W.J., Simon, G., Russo, J. *et al.* (2004) Quality of depression care in a population-based sample of patients with diabetes and major depression. *Med. Care*, **42**, 1222–1229.

23. Gary, T., Crum, R., Cooper-Patrick, L. *et al.* (2000) Depressive symptoms and metabolic control in African-Americans with type 2 diabetes. *Diabetes Care*, **23**, 23–29.

24. Thomas, J., Jones, G., Scarinci, I., and Brantley, P. (2003) A descriptive and comparative study of the prevalence of depressive and anxiety disorders in low-income adults with type 2 diabetes and other chronic illnesses. *Diabetes Care*, **26**, 2311–2317.

25. Egede, L.E. and Zheng, D. (2003) Independent factors associated with major depressive disorder in a national sample of individuals with diabetes. *Diabetes Care*, **26**, 104–111.

26. Bell, R.A., Smith, S.L., Arcury, T.A. *et al.* (2005) Prevalence and correlates of depressive symptoms among rural older African Americans, native Americans, and whites with diabetes. *Diabetes Care*, **28**, 823–829.

27. Fisher, L., Chesla, C., Mullan, J. *et al.* (2001) Contributors to depression in Latino and European-American patients with type 2 diabetes. *Diabetes Care*, **24**, 1751–1757.

28. Trief, P.M., Morin, P.C., Izquierdo, R. *et al.* (2006) Depression and glycemic control in elderly ethnically diverse patients with diabetes: The IDEATel Project. *Diabetes Care*, **29**, 830–835.

29. Asghar, S., Hussain, A., Ali, S. *et al.* (2007) Prevalence of depression and diabetes: a population-based study from rural Bangladesh. *Diabet. Med.*, **24**, 872–877.

30. Singh, P.K., Looker, H.C., Hanson, R.L. *et al.* (2004) Depression, diabetes, and glycemic control in Pima Indians. *Diabetes Care*, **27**, 618–619.

31. Zahid, N., Asghar, S., Claussen, B., and Hussain, A. (2008) Depression and diabetes in a rural community in Pakistan. *Diabetes Res. Clin. Pract.*, **79**, 124–127.

32. Pouwer, F., Skinner, T., Pibernik-Okanovic, M. *et al.* (2005) Serious diabetes-specific emotional problems and depression in a Croatian-Dutch-English survey from the European Depression in Diabetes (EDID) Research Consortium. *Diabetes Res. Clin. Pract.*, **70**, 166–173.

33. de Jonge, P., Roy, J., Saz, P. *et al.* (2006) Prevalent and incident depression in community-dwelling elderly persons with diabetes mellitus: results from the ZARADEMP project. *Diabetologia*, **49**, 2627–2633.

34. Hislop, A., Fegan, P., Schlaeppi, M. *et al.* (2008) Prevalence and associations of psychological distress in young adults with type 1 diabetes. *Diabet. Med.*, **25**, 91–96.

35. Peyrot, M. and Rubin, R.R. (1997) Levels and risks of depression and anxiety symptomatology among diabetic adults. *Diabetes Care*, **20**, 585–590.

36. Hermanns, N., Kulzer, B., Krichbaum, M. *et al.* (2005) Affective and anxiety disorders in a German sample of diabetic patients: prevalence, comorbidity and risk factors. *Diabet. Med.*, **22**, 293–300.

37. Eaton, W., Shao, H., Nestadt, G. *et al.* (2008) Population-based study of first onset and chronicity in major depressive disorder. *Arch. Gen. Psychiatry*, **65**, 513–520.

38. Brown, G.W., Bifulco, A., and Harris, T.O. (1987) Life events, vulnerability and onset of depression: some refinements. *Br. J. Psychiatry*, **50**, 30–42.

39. Kessler, R. (1997) The effects of stressful life events on depression. *Ann. Rev. Psychol.*, **48**, 191–214.

40. Kendler, K.S., Karkowski, L.M., and Prescott, C.A. (1999) Causal relationship between stressful life events and the onset of major depression. *Am. J. Psychiatry*, **156**, 837–841.
41. Carvalhais, S., Lima-Costa, M., Peixoto, S. *et al.* (2008) The influence of socio-economic conditions on the prevalence of depressive symptoms and its covariates in an elderly population with slight income differences: the Bambuí Health and Aging Study (BHAS). *Int. J. Soc. Psychiatry*, **54**, 447–456.
42. Pilowsky, D., Wickramaratne, P., Rush, A. *et al.* (2006) Children of currently depressed mothers: a STAR*D ancillary study. *J. Clin. Psychiatry*, **67**, 126–136.
43. Jaser, S.S., Whittemore, R., Ambrosino, J.M. *et al.* (2008) Mediators of depressive symptoms in children with type 1 diabetes and their mothers. *J. Pediatr. Psychol.*, **33**, 509–519.
44. Thompson, C., Syddall, H., Rodin, I. *et al.* (2001) Birth weight and the risk of depressive disorder in late life. *Br. J. Psychiatry*, **179**, 450–455.
45. Paile-Hyvärinen, M., Räikkönen, K., Forsén, T. *et al.* (2007) Depression and its association with diabetes, cardiovascular disease, and birth weight. *Ann. Med.*, **39**, 634–640.
46. Lustman, P., Griffith, L., and Clouse, R. (1988) Depression in adults with diabetes. Results of 5-yr follow-up study. *Diabetes Care*, **11**, 605–612.
47. Brooks, R.J. (1999) Gender differences in the effect of the subjective experience of diabetes and sense of control on distress. *Health*, **3**, 399–421.
48. Lewinsohn, P., Rohde, P., Seeley, J., and Fischer, S. (1991) Age and depression: unique and shared effects. *Psychol. Aging*, **6**, 247–260.
49. Roberts, R., Kaplan, G., Shema, S., and Strawbridge, W. (1997) Does growing old increase the risk for depression? *Am. J. Psychiatry*, **154**, 1384–1390.
50. Mast, B., Miles, T., Penninx, B. *et al.* (2008) Vascular disease and future risk of depressive symptomatology in older adults: findings from the Health, Aging, and Body Composition study. *Biol. Psychiatry*, **64**, 320–326.
51. Collins, M.M., Corcoran, P., and Perry, J. (2009) Anxiety and depression symptoms in patients with diabetes. *Diabet. Med.*, **26**, 153–161.
52. Fisher, L., Skaff, M.M., Mullan, J.T. *et al.* (2008) A longitudinal study of affective and anxiety disorders, depressive affect and diabetes distress in adults with type 2 diabetes. *Diabet. Med.*, **25**, 1096–1101.
53. Kovacs, M., Obrosky, D.S., Goldston, D., and Drash, A. (1997) Major depressive disorder in youths with IDDM: a controlled prospective study of course and outcome. *Diabetes Care*, **20**, 45–51.

54. Peyrot, M. and Rubin, R.R. (1999) Persistence of depressive symptoms in diabetic adults. *Diabetes Care*, **22,** 448–452.

55. Lustman, P.J., Griffith, L.S., Freedland, K.E., and Clouse, R.E. (1997) The course of major depression in diabetes. *Gen. Hosp. Psychiatry*, **19,** 138–143.

56. Simpson, H., Nee, J., and Endicott, J. (1997) First-episode major depression. Few sex differences in course. *Arch. Gen. Psychiatry*, **54,** 633–639.

57. Post, R.M. (1992) Transduction of psychosocial stress into the neurobiology of recurrent affective disorder. *Am. J. Psychiatry*, **149,** 999–1010.

58. Stroud, C., Davila, J., and Moyer, A. (2008) The relationship between stress and depression in first onsets versus recurrences: a meta-analytic review. *J. Abnorm. Psychol.*, **117,** 206–213.

59. Monroe, S.M., Slowich, G.M., Torres, L.D., and Gotlib, I.H. (2007) Major life events and major chronic difficulties are differentially associated with history of major depressive episodes. *J. Abnorm. Psychol.*, **116,** 116–124.

60. Kendler, K.S., Thornton, L.M., and Gardner, C.O. (2000) Stressful life events and previous episodes in the etiology of major depression in women: an evaluation of the "kindling" hypothesis. *Am. J. Psychiatry*, **157,** 1243–1251.

61. Monroe, S. and Harkness, K. (2005) Life stress, the "kindling" hypothesis, and the recurrence of depression: considerations from a life stress perspective. *Psychol. Rev.*, **112,** 417–445.

62. Bruce, D., Casey, G., Davis, W. *et al.* (2006) Vascular depression in older people with diabetes. *Diabetologia*, **49,** 2828–2836.

63. de Groot, M., Anderson, R.M., Freedland, K.E. *et al.* (2001) Association of depression and diabetes complications: a meta-analysis. *Psychosom. Med.*, **63,** 619–630.

64. Katon, W., Russo, J., Lin, E.H.B. *et al.* (2009) Depression and diabetes: factors associated with major depression at five-year follow-up. *Psychosomatics*, **50,** 570–579.

65. Knol, M., Heerdink, F., Egberts, A. *et al.* (2007) Depressive symptoms in subjects with diagnosed and undiagnosed type 2 diabetes. *Psychosom. Med.*, **69,** 300–305.

66. Palinkas, L., Barrett-Connor, E., and Wingard, D. (1991) Type 2 diabetes and depressive symptoms in older adults: a population-based study. *Diabet. Med.*, **8,** 532–539.

67. Icks, A., Kruse, J., Dragano, N. *et al.* (2008) Are symptoms of depression more common in diabetes? Results from the Heinz Nixdorf Recall study. *Diabet. Med.*, **25,** 1330–1336.

68. Padgett, D.K. (1993) Sociodemographic and disease-related correlates of depressive morbidity among diabetic patients in Zagreb, Croatia. *J. Nerv. Ment. Dis.*, **181**, 123–129.

69. Bruce, D.G., Davis, W.A., and Davis, T.M.E. (2005) Longitudinal predictors of reduced mobility and physical disability in patients with type 2 diabetes. *Diabetes Care*, **28**, 2441–2447.

70. Wikblad, K., Wibell, L., and Montin, K. (1991) Health and unhealth in chronic disease. *Scand. J. Caring Sci.*, **5**, 71–77.

71. Pawaskar, M., Anderson, R., and Balkrishnan, R. (2007) Self-reported predictors of depressive symptomatology in an elderly population with type 2 diabetes mellitus: a prospective cohort study. *Health & Quality of Life Outcomes*, **5**, 50.

72. Lysy, Z., Da Costa, D., and Dasgupta, K. (2008) The association of physical activity and depression in Type 2 diabetes. *Diabet. Med.*, **25**, 1133–1341.

73. Anstey, K., von Sanden, C., Sargent-Cox, K., and Luszcz, M. (2007) Prevalence and risk factors for depression in a longitudinal, population-based study including individuals in the community and residential care. *Am. J. Geriatr. Psychiatry*, **15**, 497–501.

74. Fitten, L., Ortiz, F., Fairbanks, L. *et al.* (2008) Depression, diabetes and metabolic-nutritional factors in elderly Hispanics. *J. Nutr. Health Aging*, **12**, 634–640.

75. Luijendijk, H., Stricker, B., Hofman, A. *et al.* (2008) Cerebrovascular risk factors and incident depression in community-dwelling elderly. *Acta Psychiatr. Scand.*, **118**, 139–148.

76. Moreira, R.O., Marca, K.F., Appolinario, J.C., and Coutinho, W.F. (2007) Increased waist circumference is associated with an increased prevalence of mood disorders and depressive symptoms in obese women. *Eat. Weight Disord.*, **12**, 35–40.

77. Polonsky, W., Anderson, B., Lohrer, P. *et al.* (1995) Assessment of diabetes related distress. *Diabetes Care*, **18**, 754–760.

78. Black, S.A. (1999) Increased health burden associated with comorbid depression in older diabetic Mexican Americans. Results from the Hispanic Established Population for the Epidemiologic Study of the Elderly Survey. *Diabetes Care*, **22**, 56–64.

79. Palinkas, L., Lee, P., and Barrett-Connor, E. (2004) A prospective study of Type 2 diabetes and depressive symptoms in the elderly: the Rancho Bernardo Study. *Diabet. Med.*, **21**, 1185–1191.

80. Polsky, D., Doshi, J., Marcus, S. *et al.* (2005) Long-term risk for depressive symptoms after a medical diagnosis. *Arch. Intern. Med.*, **165**, 1260–1266.

81. Golden, S., Lazo, M., Carnethon, M. *et al.* (2008) Examining a bidirectional association between depressive symptoms and diabetes. *JAMA*, **299**, 2751–2759.

82. Brown, L., Majumdar, S., Newman, S., and Johnson, J. (2006) Type 2 diabetes does not increase risk of depression. *Can. Med. Assoc. J.*, **175**, 42–46.

83. Engum, A. (2007) The role of depression and anxiety in onset of diabetes in a large population-based study. *J. Psychosom. Res.*, **62**, 31–38.

84. Kim, J.M., Stewart, R., Kim, S.W. *et al.* (2006) Vascular risk factors and incident late-life depression in a Korean population. *Br. J. Psychiatry*, **189**, 26–30.

85. Mezuk, B., Eaton, W.W., Albrecht, S., and Golden, S.H. (2008) Depression and Type 2 diabetes over the lifespan: a meta-analysis. *Diabetes Care*, **31**, 2383–2390.

86. Willis, T. (1674) *Pharmaceutice Rationalis Sive Diatriba De Medicamentorum Operationibus in Humano Corpore*, Theatro Sheldoniano, Oxford.

87. Knol, M.J., Twisk, J.W.R., Beekman, A.T.F. *et al.* (2006) Depression as a risk factor for the onset of type 2 diabetes mellitus. A meta-analysis. *Diabetologia*, **49**, 837–845.

88. Van der Kooy, K., van Hout, H., Marwijk, H. *et al.* (2007) Depression and the risk for cardiovascular diseases: systematic review and meta analysis. *Int. J. Geriatr. Psychiatry*, **22**, 613–626.

89. Whooley, M.A., de Jonge, P., Vittinghoff, E. *et al.* (2008) Depressive symptoms, health behaviors and risk of cardiovascular events in patients with coronary heart disease. *JAMA*, **300**, 2379–2388.

90. Brown, E.S., Varghese, F.P., and McEwen, B.S. (2004) Association of depression with medical illness: does cortisol play a role? *Biol. Psychiatry*, **55**, 1–9.

91. Vogelzangs, N., Kritchevsky, S.B., Beekman, A.T.F. *et al.* (2008) Depressive symptoms and change in abdominal obesity in older persons. *Arch. Gen. Psychiatry*, **65**, 1386–1393.

92. Hu, J., Amoako, E.P., Gruber, K.J., and Rossen, E.K. (2007) The relationship among health functioning indicators and depression in older adults with diabetes. *Issues Ment. Health Nurs.*, **28**, 133–150.

93. Manson, J., Rimm, E., Stampfer, M. *et al.* (1991) Physical activity and incidence of non-insulin-dependent diabetes mellitus in women. *Lancet*, **338**, 774–778.

94. UK Prospective Diabetes Study (UKPDS) Group (1998) Intensive blood-glucose control with sulphonylureas or insulin compared with

conventional treatment and risk of complications in patients with type 2 diabetes. *Lancet*, **352**, 837–853.

95. The Diabetes Control and Complications Trial Research Group (1993) The effect of intensive treatment of diabetes on the development and progression of long-term complications in insulin-dependent diabetes mellitus. *N. Engl. J. Med.*, **329**, 977–985.

96. Ciechanowski, P.S., Katon, W.J., and Russo, J.E. (2000) Depression and diabetes: impact of depressive symptoms on adherence, function and costs. *Arch. Intern. Med.*, **160**, 3278–3285.

97. Hampson, S., Glasgow, R., and Strycker, L. (2000) Beliefs versus feelings: a comparison of personal models and depression for predicting multiple outcomes in diabetes. *Br. J. Health Psychol.*, **5**, 27–29.

98. Katon, W., Russo, J., Lin, E.H.B. *et al.* (2009) Diabetes and poor disease control: is depression associated with poor adherence or lack of treatment intensification? *Psychosom. Med.*, **71**, 965–972.

99. Lustman, P.J., Anderson, R.J., Freedland, K.E. *et al.* (2000) Depression and poor glycemic control. A meta-analytic review of the literature. *Diabetes Care*, **23**, 934–942.

100. Katon, W.J., Rutter, C., Simon, G. *et al.* (2005) The association of comorbid depression with mortality in patients with type 2 diabetes. *Diabetes Care*, **28**, 2668–2672.

101. Ismail, K., Winkley, K., Stahl, D. *et al.* (2007) A cohort study of people with diabetes and their first foot ulcer: the role of depression on mortality. *Diabetes Care*, **30**, 1473–1479.

102. Nakahara, R., Yoshiuchi, K., Kumano, H. *et al.* (2006) Prospective study on influence of psychosocial factors on glycemic control in Japanese patients with type 2 diabetes. *Psychosomatics*, **47**, 240–246.

103. Richardson, L.K., Egede, L.E., Mueller, M. *et al.* (2008) Longitudinal effects of depression on glycemic control in veterans with Type 2 diabetes. *Gen. Hosp. Psychiatry*, **30**, 509–514.

104. Lustman, P.J., Clouse, R.E., Freedland, K.E. *et al.* (1997) Effects of nortriptyline on depression and glucose regulation in diabetes: results of a double-blind placebo-controlled trial. *Psychosom. Med.*, **59**, 241–250.

105. Lustman, P., Freedland, K., Griffith, L., and Clouse, R. (2000) Fluoxetine for depression in diabetes: a randomized double-blind placebo-controlled trial. *Diabetes Care*, **23**, 618–623.

106. Lustman, P.J., Clouse, R.E., Nix, B.D. *et al.* (2006) Sertraline for prevention of depression recurrence in diabetes mellitus. *Arch. Gen. Psychiatry*, **63**, 521–529.

107. Paile-Hyvärinen, M., Wahlbeck, K., and Eriksson, J. (2003) Quality of life and metabolic status in mildly depressed women with type 2 diabetes treated with paroxetine: a single-blind randomised placebo controlled trial. *BMC Fam. Pract.*, **4,** 7.

108. Katon, W., Von Korff, M., Ciechanowski, P. *et al.* (2004) Behavioral and clinical factors associated with depression among individuals with diabetes. *Diabetes Care*, **27,** 914–920.

109. Williams, J.W., Katon, W., Lin, E.H.B. *et al.* (2004) The effectiveness of depression care management on diabetes-related outcomes in older patients. *Ann. Intern. Med.*, **140,** 1015–1024.

110. Aikens, J. and Piette, J.D. (2009) Diabetic patients' medication under-use, illness outcomes, and beliefs about antihyperglycemic and antihypertensive treatments. *Diabetes Care*, **32,** 1177–1181.

111. McCarthy, M. (1990) The thin ideal, depression and eating disorders in women. *Behav. Res. Ther.*, **28,** 205–214.

112. Bryden, K.S., Peveler, R.C., Stein, A. *et al.* (2001) Clinical and psychological course of diabetes from adolescence to young adulthood. *Diabetes Care*, **24,** 1536–1540.

113. Rydall, A.C., Rodin, G.M., Olmstead, M.P. *et al.* (1997) Disordered eating behavior and microvascular complications in young women with insulin-dependent diabetes mellitus. *N. Engl. J. Med.*, **336,** 1849–1854.

114. Jones, J.M., Lawson, M.L., Daneman, D. *et al.* (2000) Eating disorders in adolescent females with and without type 1 diabetes: cross sectional study. *BMJ*, **320,** 1563–1566.

115. Colton, P., Olmstead, M.P., Daneman, D. *et al.* (2004) Disturbed eating behavior and eating disorders in preteen and early teenage girls with type 1 diabetes. *Diabetes Care*, **27,** 1654–1659.

116. Grigsby, A.B., Anderson, R.J., Freedland, K.E. *et al.* (2002) Prevalence of anxiety in adults with diabetes: a systematic review. *J. Psychosom. Res.*, **53,** 1053–1060.

117. Mollema, E.D., Snoek, F.J., Adér, H.J. *et al.* (2001) Insulin-treated diabetes patients with fear of self-injecting or fear of self-testing: psychological comorbidity and general well-being. *J. Psychosom. Res.*, **51,** 665–672.

118. Snoek, F., Mollema, E., Heine, R. *et al.* (1997) Development and validation of the Diabetes Fear of Injecting and Self-Testing Questionnaire (D-FISQ): first findings. *Diabet. Med.*, **14,** 871–876.

119. Karlson, B. and Agardh, C.D. (1997) Burden of illness, metabolic control and complications in relation to depressive symptoms in IDDM patients. *Diabet. Med.*, **14,** 1066–1072.

120. Polonsky, W.H., Fisher, L., Guzman, S. *et al.* (2005) Psychological insulin resistance in patients with Type 2 diabetes: the scope of the problem. *Diabetes Care*, **28**, 2543–2545.

121. Petrak, F., Stridde, E., Leverkus, F. *et al.* (2007) Development and validation of a new measure to evaluate psychological resistance to insulin treatment. *Diabetes Care*, **30**, 2199–2204.

122. Pibernik-Okanović, M., Begić, D., Peroš, K. *et al.* (2008) Psychosocial factors contributing to persistent depressive symptoms in type 2 diabetic patients: a Croatian survey from the European Depression in Diabetes Research Consortium. *J. Diabetes Comp.*, **22**, 246–253.

123. Lin, E.H.B., Katon, W., Von Korff, M. *et al.* (2004) Relationship of depression and diabetes self-care, medication adherence, and preventive care. *Diabetes Care*, **27**, 2154–2160.

124. Wade, A.N., Farmer, A.J., and French, D.P. (2004) Association of beliefs about illness and medication with self-care activities in non-insulin treated Type 2 diabetes. *Diabetes Care*, **21**(Suppl.), 52.

125. Skinner, T.C., Hampson, S.E., and Fife-Schaw, C. (2002) Personality, personal model beliefs and self-care in adolescents and young adults with Type 1 diabetes. *Health Psychol.*, **21**, 61–70.

126. Heller, S., Davies, M.J., Khunti, K. *et al.* (2005) The illness beliefs of people newly diagnosed with type 2 diabetes: results from the DESMOND pilot study. *Diabetologia*, **48**(Suppl.), A324.

127. Lloyd, C.E., Wing, R.R., Matthews, K.M., and Orchard, T.J. (1992) Psychosocial factors and the complications of insulin-dependent diabetes mellitus: the Pittsburgh Epidemiology of Diabetes Complications Study – VIII. *Diabetes Care*, **15**, 166–172.

128. Orchard, T.J., Olson, J.C., Erbey, J.R. *et al.* (2003) Insulin resistance-related factors, but not glycemia, predict coronary artery disease in type 1 diabetes: 10-year follow-up data from the Pittsburgh Epidemiology of Diabetes Complications Study. *Diabetes Care*, **26**, 1374–1379.

129. Kovacs, M., Mukerji, P., Drash, A., and Iyengar, S. (1995) Biomedical and psychiatric risk factors for retinopathy among children with IDDM. *Diabetes Care*, **18**, 1592–1599.

130. Lett, H.S., Blumenthal, J.A., Babyak, M.A. *et al.* (2004) Depression is a risk factor for coronary artery disease: evidence mechanisms, and treatment. *Psychosom. Med.*, **66**, 305–315.

131. Thomas, A.J., Kalaria, R.N., and O'Brien, J.T. (2004) Depression and vascular disease: what is the relationship? *J. Affect. Disord.*, **79**, 81–95.

132. Zhang, X., Norris, S.L., Gregg, E.W. *et al.* (2005) Depressive symptoms and mortality among persons with and without diabetes. *Am. J. Epidemiol.*, **161**, 652–660.

133. Lin, E.H.B., Heckbert, S.R., Rutter, C.M. *et al.* (2009) Depression and increased mortality in diabetes: unexpected causes of death. *Ann. Family Med.*, **7**, 414–421.

134. Black, S.A., Markides, K.S., and Ray, L.A. (2003) Depression predicts increased incidence of adverse health outcomes in older Mexican Americans with type 2 diabetes. *Diabetes Care*, **26**, 2822–2828.

135. Evans, J., MacDonald, T., Leese, G. *et al.* (2000) Impact of type 1 and type 2 diabetes on patterns and costs of drug prescribing: a population-based study. *Diabetes Care*, **23**, 770–774.

136. Everson, S., Maty, S., Lynch, J., and Kaplan, G. (2002) Epidemiologic evidence for the relation between socioeconomic status and depression, obesity, and diabetes. *J. Psychosom. Res.*, **53**, 891–895.

137. Riolo, S.A., Nguyen, T.A., and King, C.A. (2005) Prevalence of depression by race/ethnicity: findings from the National Health and Nutrition Examination Survey III. *Am. J. Public Health*, **95**, 998–1000.

# CHAPTER 2

# Unraveling the Pathogenesis of the Depression–Diabetes Link

### Khalida Ismail

*Department of Psychological Medicine, Institute of Psychiatry,
King's College London, London, UK*

The mechanisms underlying the high rates of depression in diabetes and its adverse effects on diabetes-related outcomes are not yet well understood, but are likely to include biological and psychological factors and processes that interact with each other. The aim of this chapter is to introduce the reader to a greater understanding of the potential biological mechanisms that may explain the depression–diabetes link.

The chapter focuses mainly on evidence that pertains to type 2 diabetes, unless otherwise specified. Firstly, a brief overview of the limitations of a pure psychological model to explain the higher prevalence of depression in people with diabetes and the adverse effects of depression on diabetes outcomes are given. This is followed by a synthesis of the evidence for potential biological processes in which depression is associated with metabolic dysfunction; these include the association between depression and insulin resistance, which is the beginning of the diabetes continuum, and the pathways that might mediate this association, such as the hypothalamic–pituitary–adrenal

*Depression and Diabetes*  Edited by Wayne Katon, Mario Maj and Norman Sartorius
© 2010 John Wiley & Sons, Ltd

(HPA) axis, the innate immune response and the autonomic nervous system. The difficulties in studying the direction(s) of the cause and effect of the association are highlighted. Thirdly, the notion that depression and diabetes may have common origins is explored by examining evidence from life course epidemiology, such as common genetic vulnerability, foetal nutrition and childhood adversity. The little understood metabolic and immune effects of antidepressants are briefly reviewed.

Finally, this theoretical complex multifactorial model is summarized, with a view to future directions. As further insights into this rapidly emerging field develop, this could ultimately lead to novel targets for primary prevention and treatments for diabetes and/or depression.

## LIMITATIONS OF THE PSYCHOLOGICAL MODEL

The psychological model has been the conventional explanation for the association between depression and diabetes, namely that the emotional and practical burden related to diabetes is the predisposing factor for depression. In other words, depression is a consequence of diabetes. Depression moderates lifestyle behaviours such as diet and weight, physical activity and smoking [1–3]. Depression is associated with reduced diabetes self-care behaviours [4–6] and this has been substantiated in recent prospective studies [7, 8].

The psychological model, however, does not fully account for the adverse effects of depression. Others have argued that the direction of the association is reversed, or bilateral, as depression appears to be present before the onset of diabetes [9, 10]. The adverse effects of depression on diabetes outcomes cannot be solely explained by its mediating effects on reducing diabetes self-care, which would be expected to translate into poor glycaemic control and complications. The association between depression and glycaemic control is small in cross-sectional studies [11, 12] and almost disappears in most of the handful of prospective studies [13–18]. In addition, there is little evidence at present from randomized controlled trials that treating depression alone in diabetes improves glycaemic control, although the treatments do improve mood [19]. Some investigators have proposed that diabetes-specific thoughts, worries and feelings, in other words diabetes distress, are a more important prognostic factor for reduced self-care than the cognitive, affective and behavioural correlates of depression, although clearly the two are not mutually exclusive psychological processes [16].

Similar limitations of the psychological model have also been observed in people with depression and coronary artery disease (CAD), which is relevant as type 2 diabetes and cardiovascular diseases share a common causal pathway [20]. Depression is also associated with increased mortality rates in people with CAD [21–24], yet appears to explain only a third of the variance in adherence to cardiovascular medication [25]. Further, in randomized controlled trials of treatments (antidepressants, psychotherapy or combinations) for depression in people who have had acute cardiac events, mood tends to improve, but there is no significant improvement in cardiovascular outcomes [26, 27]. This suggests that additional mechanisms, such as biological processes, need to be considered to help explain the depression–diabetes link (Figure 2.1).

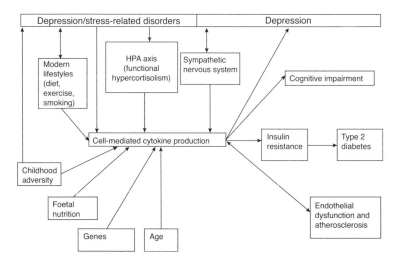

**Figure 2.1**   A schematic diagram of theoretical mechanisms that explain the depression–diabetes link.

## DEPRESSION AND INSULIN RESISTANCE

The diabetes continuum stretches from insulin resistance to impaired glucose tolerance and frank diabetes as insulin secretion fails. Insulin resistance is defined as decreased sensitivity of the peripheral insulin receptors to the action of insulin. In response to this, pancreatic islet ß-cells secrete higher circulating levels of insulin to compensate for the reduced peripheral receptor function. Insulin resistance is measured by the degree to which glucose is cleared from the blood in response to a given amount of insulin in the fasting state. Insulin resistance was considered to be only at peripheral sites, such as adipose tissue, but, as glucose and insulin cross the blood–brain barrier, the notion of central insulin resistance is emerging. The insulin receptors in the brain have a different structure and function to those in the periphery, but there is accumulating evidence that peripheral insulin resistance is associated with functional decline in the central nervous system [28] and could be a causal link to Alzheimer's dementia and vascular dementia. Insulin resistance is also a determinant of free fatty acids in the blood, which are in turn important in tryptophan metabolism and brain serotonin concentrations. Physical inactivity and obesity, both behaviours mediated by depression, lead to insulin resistance. These are just some of the observations that point to a putative biological link to depression.

There is now a small and slowly growing body of epidemiological studies examining the association between depression and insulin resistance (Table 2.1). One of the earliest first observational studies was the British Women's Heart and Health study of 4286 women aged 60–79 years randomly selected from primary care. The association between depression and glucose dysregulation was almost U-shaped, with the prevalence of depression (measured by self-report and antidepressant prescribing) decreasing linearly with increasing insulin resistance (measured by the homeostasis model assessment method, HOMA score) among women without diabetes and increasing among women with diabetes [29]. In contrast, in a population-based study of 491 midlife to elderly Finnish participants, insulin resistance (measured by the qualitative insulin sensitivity check index, QUICKI) and severity of depressive symptoms (measured by the Beck's Depression Inventory) were positively correlated, particularly in people

**Table 2.1** Observational studies of the association between depression and insulin resistance

| Study | Design | N | Age (years) | Gender | Results |
|---|---|---|---|---|---|
| Lawlor et al. [29] | Cross-sectional | 4286 | 60–79 | Women | odds ratio = −0.84 (0.74–0.97), $p = 0.006$ |
| Everson-Rose et al. [38] | Prospective, 3 years | 2662 | 46.4 ($\pm$2.7) | Women | No difference in rate of increase in HOMA-IR per year (depression-by-time interaction, $p = 0.39$) |
| Lawlor et al. [39] | Prospective, 12 years | 2512 | 45–59 | Men | odds ratio = 0.97 (0.77–1.23), $p =$ not significant |
| Timonen et al. [30] | Cross-sectional | 491 | 71–73 | Men and women | $r = 0.13$, $p = 0.004$ |
| Adriaanse et al. [31] | Cross-sectional | 541 | 55–75 | Men and women | $r = 0.156$, $p < 0.001$ |
| Timonen et al. [34] | Cross-sectional | 2609 | 31 | Men | odds ratio = 3.15 (1.48–6.68), p for trend = 0.007 |
| Timonen et al. [33] | Cross-sectional | 1054 | 19 | Men | odds ratio = 2.8 (1.2–6.5) |
| Pan et al. [32] | Cross-sectional | 3285 | 50–70 | Men and women | odds ratio = 1.54 (1.17–2.04), $p = 0.002$ |

with impaired glucose tolerance [30]. The Finnish findings have been replicated in Dutch [31] and Chinese [32] samples of similar age groups. The strongest association was observed in young healthy Finnish male military conscripts (n = 1054), where moderate to severe depressive symptoms (measured by the modified Beck's Depression Inventory) were associated with an almost threefold risk of insulin resistance (measured by the HOMA-IR), but mild depressive symptoms were not [33]. Similar findings were observed in the young males from the Northern Finland 1966 Birth Cohort [34]. The major limitation of these studies is the use of self-report depression, which may have misclassified symptoms of undiagnosed diabetes as depressive.

There have been few studies that have examined the direction of the association between depression and diabetes. In a small but well designed case-control study from Japan, 20 non-diabetes patients with depression were compared with 13 age-, sex- and body mass index (BMI) matched non-depressed controls. Using the frequently sampled intravenous glucose tolerance test, and the oral glucose tolerance test (OGTT), depressed cases had higher insulin resistance than controls. In the depressed group, after treatment with tricyclic antidepressants while caloric intake and physical activity were controlled, there was significant improvement in insulin sensitivity without changes in the BMI or fasting blood glucose [35]. In a German double-blind randomized controlled trial comparing paroxetine with amitriptyline (n = 80) in non-diabetes inpatients with DSM-IV major depressive disorder, the insulin sensitivity index (measured using the Matsuda method) increased (in other words improved) only in those patients who remitted from major depressive disorder as a result of treatment with either antidepressant over five weeks while correcting for BMI [36]. However, these positive findings were not observed in a similarly designed sample of euglycaemic women of reproductive age [37].

The Study of Women's Health Across the Nation followed 2662 women from the main ethnic groups in the United States over three years. It found that depression (measured on the Center for Epidemiological Studies-Depression Scale score) was associated with insulin resistance (measured on the HOMA-IR), which increased by 0.05

units per year, and with a 66% increase in incident diabetes, both of which became non-significant when adjustment for central adiposity was made, except in African American women. One interpretation is that adjusting for central adiposity could be an overadjustment, as it is on the same causal pathway for insulin resistance. Depression was associated with absolute levels of the HOMA-IR, but not with changes in the HOMA-IR over time, making the interpretation of which came first difficult [38].

In the Caerphilly prospective cohort study, 2203 Welsh males in their midlife were followed up at three time points over 14 years. There was no significant prospective association between baseline insulin resistance HOMA-IR and depression over time (as measured on the 30 item General Health Questionnaire) [39].

The synthesis of the literature on the association between depression and insulin resistance is promising but not conclusive. While most of the cross-sectional studies demonstrate an association, this seems to be particularly strong in populations indigenous to the Northern Hemisphere. There have been too few prospective studies to arrive at a consensus, but the most promising research may lie in suitably matched case-control experimental settings, where the effects of multiple confounders and colinear variables can be dealt with.

## DEPRESSION AND ACTIVITY OF THE HYPOTHALAMIC–PITUITARY–ADRENAL (HPA) AXIS

The stress response (the flight–fright response) is a process that allows the body to deal with threats, whether environmental or psychological. Stress activates the HPA axis, which leads to a cascade of responses to the adverse stimuli and allows the body to return to homeostatis. Firstly, corticotropin-releasing hormone (CRH) is released onto pituitary receptors. This stimulus results in the secretion of corticotropin into plasma, which stimulates corticotropin receptors in the adrenal cortex, which results in the release of cortisol into the blood. Increased cortisol production leads to inhibition of the gonadal, growth hormone and thyroid axes (which reduces lipolysis and is anabolic) and, at physiological levels, activates the inflammatory response. The HPA axis also activates the sympathetic nervous system (SNS), which increases catecholamines (adrenaline and noradrenaline), stimulates the innate immune response, decreases neurovegetative functions (such as appetite and sleep) and heightens cognitive functioning. The collective metabolic effects are gluconeogenesis, glycogenolysis and insulin resistance [40]. Cushing's syndrome is the medical paradigm of chronic activation of the HPA axis, in which chronic hypercortisolaemia leads to multisystem effects, with hypertension, glucose dysregulation from insulin resistance to frank diabetes, lipid dysregulation, osteoporosis, myopathy and neuropsychiatric symptoms. Emerging data suggest that metabolic syndrome is linked to HPA hyperactivity, such that increased or persistent exposure to low grade or 'functional hypercortisolism' contributes to increased visceral fat accumulation [41].

The causal direction for this activation of the HPA axis remains uncertain, but may be partly associated with oxidative stress and immune response to obesity and partly to the direct effects of stress as perceived by the brain. This idea was first proposed by Bjorntorp in the early 1990s, when he purported that visceral obesity was a 'civilization' syndrome [42, 43]. The association between chronic stress states and cardiovascular disease is at least partly mediated by increased circulating cortisol levels and greater responsiveness of the HPA axis. In recent years, with the epidemic of obesity, Bjorntorp's theory has re-gained interest. Mechanization of transport and cheap fatty foods encourage sedentary lifestyles and overeating, both innate human behaviours that have been argued were evolutionary adaptations to conserve energy, as a response to stress of modern living. Obesity damages adipocytes and causes oxidative stress, which activates the HPA axis, which in turn leads to increased cortisol release and SNS stimulation, which induces the innate inflammatory response and, ultimately, insulin resistance and endothelial dysfunction.

There is a vast literature and now considerable evidence that cortisol and its central releasing factor, CRH, are involved in depression, and this has been reviewed extensively in recent years [44–47]. Briefly, mean higher free, unbound cortisol levels in the plasma, increased 24-hour urinary free cortisol secretion and elevated CRH levels in cerebrospinal fluid have been observed in depressed patients when compared to controls [48–51]. In studies using dexamethasone to evaluate the sensitivity of the hypothalamus to feedback signals for the shutdown of CRH release, the normal cortisol suppression response is absent in about half of the most severely depressed patients, and there is a dose–response association between cortisol suppression and severity of depression [48], although in larger population-based studies this finding is less strong [49]. Antidepressant-induced clinical remission is accompanied by reversal of some of these abnormalities [44]. Techniques continue to be improved, so that over time there will be a greater understanding of the complexity of cortisol dynamics [50].

Despite this vast literature, there are difficulties in establishing the causal pathways and whether aspects of HPA activity can become valid biological tests for depression. One reason is a selection bias of most studies towards severe depression, in which the association has been most strongly observed, whereas most depression in the general population is of mild to moderate severity. Secondly, there have been insufficient observational prospective studies to test the association in randomly selected or representative samples of the general population. This is partly because measuring HPA activity is cumbersome in epidemiological surveys, but there have been some recent impressive attempts.

The Heart and Soul study, which consisted of 693 outpatients with CAD, used 24-hour urinary free cortisol and assessed depression by the Computerized Diagnostic Interview Schedule [51]. The mean cortisol was higher in those with depression; those with the highest quartile of cortisol had a twofold risk for having depression compared with those in the lowest quartile, but elevated cortisol was not associated with worse cardiac function.

In a cross-sectional analysis of the Whitehall cohort, repeated measures of salivary free cortisol in 2873 healthy civil servants in the United Kingdom were inversely associated with positive affect [52].

In the Netherlands Study of Depression and Anxiety, three groups were compared: 308 control subjects without psychiatric disorders, 579 persons with remitted DSM-IV major depressive disorder, and 701 persons with a current major depressive disorder measured using the Computerized Diagnostic Interview Schedule [49]. Cortisol levels were measured in seven saliva samples to determine the one-hour cortisol awakening response, evening cortisol levels, and cortisol suppression after a 0.5 mg dexamethasone suppression test. Both the remitted and current major depressive disorder groups showed a significantly higher cortisol awakening response compared with control subjects. The post-dexamethasone cortisol level did not differ between the two major depressive disorder groups.

A third difficulty in interpreting the HPA axis data in depression is that hypercortisolaemia is not specific for depression, as there are many other factors associated with HPA activity, such as age, gender (and in women, menstrual history), time of day, acute stressors such as mental stress, life events, physical exertion and acute illnesses, heritability, smoking and a wide range of medications [53–57].

The recurrent observation that depression is not the only psychiatric disorder associated with HPA hyperactivity has led to the notion that there is a spectrum of stress reactive phenotypes that have a shared pathophysiology. The HPA axis activation in psychiatric disorders is probably a non-specific response to stress, as it has been observed in some studies of post-traumatic stress disorder [58] and chronic fatigue syndrome [59]. It is also found in schizophrenia, which may reflect the non-specific stressor effects of acute psychosis [60, 61]. Childhood adversity, such as sexual abuse and physical abuse, is associated with increased HPA activity in adult life independent of adult depression [62], but also with increased risk of depression. Furthermore, HPA activity appears to mediate the effects of early adversity on the development of chronic fatigue syndrome in adults [63], but the same pattern has not been consistently seen in studies on depressive disorders in adult life [49].

There have been few studies examining the direction of the association between depression and activation of HPA axis. Harris *et al.* [64] found that, in a primary care sample of 116 women vulnerable to depression, those with higher mean morning salivary free cortisol levels were more likely to develop depression over 13 months. Similar observations have been reported in adolescents at high risk of depression [65]. There is some evidence that hypercortisolaemic depression is associated with increased risk for CAD [66, 67].

No studies have specifically examined this association prospectively in depressed and non-depressed samples with diabetes or at high risk of diabetes, such as people with obesity or first-degree relatives of diabetes patients [68].

So, an extensive body of research demonstrates that HPA axis activation appears to be linked to the depression diathesis, although evidence of its specificity to depression is poor and the causal direction has yet to be substantiated in large scale observational studies.

## THE DIABETES–DEPRESSION LINK AND THE AUTONOMIC NERVOUS SYSTEM

The sympathetic and parasympathetic divisions of the autonomic nervous system function antagonistically to preserve a dynamic modulation of vital functions. The SNS innervates the accelerating centre of the heart, the lungs (increased ventilation and dilatation of the bronchi) and the non-striated muscles (artery contraction). It releases adrenaline and noradrenaline. The parasympathetic system innervates the cardiomoderator centre of the heart, the lungs (slower ventilatory rhythm and contraction of the bronchi) and the non-striated muscles (artery dilatation). It uses acetylcholine as its neurotransmitter.

The SNS is activated by the HPA axis during stress to produce the acute anxiety response (Figure 2.1). It has been suggested that excessive or persistent activation may lead to irregular sympathetic tone, elevated catecholamine levels and inflammatory processes, which in turn will contribute to dysfunction in various metabolic parameters. Heart rate variability (HRV) is a measure of cardiac vagal tone and is a sensitive indicator of both how well the central nervous system regulates the autonomic nervous system, and of the feedback process from peripheral neurons to the central nervous systems. HRV measures are derived by estimating the variation among a set of temporally ordered interbeat intervals, and decreased HRV is a well known risk factor for cardiac disease, arrhythmias and sudden death. Interpretability of serial HRV testing is highly dependent on accurate, precise and reproducible procedures that use established physiological manoeuvres, not dissimilar to the interpretation of data on HPA activity.

Much of the interest in HRV and depression has been in cardiovascular disease [69]. Decreased HRV has been well documented to be associated with depression [70–72] (although it has been difficult to separate the confounding effects of antidepressants, especially tricyclics, which are well known to suppress autonomic function) after myocardial infarction [21, 73], in stable CAD [74] and after coronary artery bypass surgery, suggesting that acute alterations in cardiac autonomic tone may contribute to the increased risk of CAD events and mortality in patients with depression. There have been few prospective studies, so whether HRV is a clinical predictor of worse depression or an epiphenomenon of progressive CAD is yet to be clarified.

The link of HRV with diabetes has been so far undeservedly understudied, considering that the most common causes of death in type 2 diabetes are CAD related, and that type 2 diabetes and atherosclerosis are related processes [20, 69]. In particular, autonomic neuropathy is a serious and common complication of diabetes. Its prevalence varies depending on the selection criteria of the study, but in randomly selected samples of people with asymptomatic diabetes, approximately 20% had abnormal cardiovascular autonomic function, which can be present within the first year of diagnosis [75]. It tends to go unrecognized, partly because it frequently coexists with other diabetes complications, especially other peripheral neuropathies, which clinically often take precedent if they are painful.

Autonomic neuropathy has multisystem and multiorgan expressions, such as cardiovascular autonomic neuropathy, which manifests as resting tachycardia, exercise intolerance, orthostatic or postural hypotension, and decreased HRV. It is associated with a twofold increased risk of silent myocardial ischemia and mortality [75]. Other manifestations include sudomotor dysfunction, which leads to loss of sweating and dry skin with consequent infections and ulcerations, impaired neurovascular function, hypoglycaemic autonomic failure, gastrointestinal effects including gastroparesis, constipation and/or diarrhea, bladder and sexual (males and females) dysfunction. The assessment of the presence of autonomic neuropathy is usually based on a battery of autonomic function tests rather than just on one test.

Studies examining whether autonomic neuropathy is linked to the association between depression and diabetes are almost non-existent. The limited literature is related to gastrointestinal symptoms (not

HRV), whose pathogenesis is controversial but in which autonomic neuropathy is considered a likely differential. In a study from Australia in a consecutive sample of outpatients with diabetes mellitus (n = 209) and a random sample of community diabetics (n = 892), the mean anxiety and depression (Hospital Anxiety and Depression Scale) and neuroticism (Eysenck short neuroticism scale) scores were significantly higher for most gastrointestinal symptoms, even after adjusting for age, gender, duration and type of diabetes, and self-reported glycaemic control [76]. This is a difficult study to interpret, but it seems to be in keeping with observations from larger cross-sectional studies that, among patients with diabetes, those with major depression report nearly twice as many diabetes symptoms than those without depression, even after adjusting for demographic characteristics, objective measures of diabetes severity and medical comorbidity [77].

It seems plausible that, if depression is linked to reduced HRV in CAD, it may also be linked to autonomic neuropathy in diabetes. At present, the data are too limited to make any conclusion about whether this association, if it exists in diabetes, is cause or effect, coincidence or colinear in progressive diabetes. This should be a new frontier of research, as it will contribute to a greater understanding of the various mechanistic pathways from activation of the HPA axis to mortality and their implications as novel targets for intervention. It is suggested that more prospective cohort studies be undertaken of large diabetes samples that include measures of autonomic function and, in particular, compare prospectively groups with and without depression.

## THE DIABETES–DEPRESSION LINK AND THE INNATE INFLAMMATORY RESPONSE

Another potential explanation for the diabetes–depression link is that depression is associated with a cytokine-induced acute-phase response, a biologically plausible hypothesis first proposed in 1991 as 'the macrophage theory of depression' [78]. This is relevant because the acute-phase response is also closely involved in the pathogenesis of type 2 diabetes and its associated clinical and biochemical features, another hypothesis that was first proposed by Pickup and Crook in 1998 [79] and recently updated [20, 80].

The innate immune system is the body's first line of defence against environmental threats, in which pro-inflammatory cytokines – particularly interleukin (IL)-6, IL-1 and tumor necrosis factor (TNF)-$\alpha$ – are released by macrophages and other cells, and, in turn, stimulate the 'acute-phase response'. This is characterized by large changes in the concentration of blood proteins such as C-reactive protein (CRP), serum amyloid A, haptoglobulin and fibrinogen. The general purpose of the acute-phase response is to help restore homeostasis. Cytokines, such as adinopectin, IL-4 and IL-10, are anti-inflammatory and lower in both type 2 diabetes and depression [20, 80].

Overeating and underactivity cause obesity, which leads to pro-inflammatory cytokine production from adipocytes and from the macrophages that accumulate in fat tissue. Cytokines act on the brain to cause behavioural changes that may manifest as depressive symptoms. The HPA axis and SNS activate the immune response, and cytokines have a feedback effect, further stimulating the HPA axis and the SNS. This, in turn, leads to increased cortisol and laying down of visceral fat.

Production of pro-inflammatory cytokines and the acute-phase response are also associated with pancreatic ß-cell apoptosis, reduced insulin secretion, insulin resistance, onset of type 2 diabetes and worse cardiovascular prognosis [81–83]. Serum sialic acid, an aggregate acute-phase response, is more strongly associated with cardiovascular mortality than glycaemic control [84].

The diabetogenic effects of the acute-phase response have led to novel interventions to improve diabetes control: a recent randomized controlled trial found that a recombinant IL-1 receptor antagonist (IL-1ra), anakinra, was effective in reducing HbA1c levels by nearly 0.5% compared to placebo, as well as reducing IL-6 and CRP levels [85, 86]. Lifestyle interventions are known to reduce the risk of type 2 diabetes, and this may be in part due to the fact that they reduce the innate inflammatory response [87].

There is growing evidence that the acute-phase response is also associated with depression. Psychological stress also causes pro-inflammatory cytokine release, because noradrenaline and CRF stimulate macrophages to release IL-6 and TNF-$\alpha$. A recent systematic review summarized the current evidence for the cross-sectional correlation between CRP, IL-1, 1L-1ra and IL-6 and depression in the general population, and in people with cancer and heart disease [88]. Overall, small to moderate associations were found between depression and CRP ($d = 0.15$), IL-6 ($d = 0.25$), IL-1 ($d = 0.35$) and IL-1ra ($d = 0.25$). The associations were stronger in those with clinical depression compared with community samples. Those studies that used clinical interviews versus self-report measures of depression were observed to have stronger associations. BMI was an important confounder, as obesity itself is related to changes in cytokines, but adjusting for other confounders, such as increasing age, sex, use of statins, antidepressants and anti-inflammatory agents, gave inconsistent results. In the handful of studies of people with CAD, depression had only a small association with CRP ($d = 0.18$) and IL-6 ($d = 0.10$) and there were no studies that measured IL-1. Measuring different inflammatory markers seems to be important, as the above review suggests that they have different associations with depression [89].

Two well-designed prospective studies have found that stress and adversity in childhood were associated with higher levels of CRP [90, 91], taking into account a wide range of biological, psychological and social confounders and associated factors. In the limited prospective studies of those with CAD, depression was correlated with levels of inflammatory markers and both variables were associated with worse cardiac outcome [92, 93].

There has been one cross-sectional study in diabetes which found that patients with depressive symptoms, compared with those who were not depressed, had only slightly higher IL-6 (median 1.3 versus 1.1 pg/ml, respectively) and CRP (median 2.2 versus 1.7 mg/l, respectively) levels [94]. The questionnaire was self-report and only two inflammatory markers were tested.

There have been no prospective studies in diabetes, and the scope for examining whether depression has a synergistic effect on the inflammatory response in diabetes is large. This is particularly of interest because of the recent development of anti-inflammatory agents which improve metabolic status. Whether they may also have an effect on mood is yet to be discovered [95].

## GENETICS OF THE DIABETES–DEPRESSION LINK

Major depression and type 2 diabetes have genetic traits that aggregate in families and this is due to a complex interaction between genetic risk and the environment. The sibling recurrence risk ratio for type 2 diabetes, a measure of the familial aggregation of the disease, has been estimated to be approximately 3 in European populations [96] and similar relative risks have been reported for major depression [97].

A recent review listed all the current candidate genes [98] that are implicated in the regulation of the HPA axis, inflammatory and serotonergic pathways. Although there has been a lot of focus on one set of stress genes, namely inflammatory genes, as they pertain to CAD and diabetes, and another set, namely serotonin genes, as they pertain to depression, in very recent years the tide has turned and more attention is being paid to the role of inflammatory genes on depression and related stress disorders. This seems particularly pertinent, as a recent meta-analysis concluded that the most well-known candidate gene for depression, the short allele polymorphism of the serotonin transporter gene (5-HTTLPR), was not, in pooled data, associated with increased risk of depression [99]. This review, which attracted some criticism from the field, appears to refute earlier promising observations that the short allele was associated with higher mean 24-hour noradrenaline excretion among those with CAD [100], and with higher mean morning cortisol levels in adolescents at high risk for depression [56].

In the first published twin study that considered depression and CAD together, the correlation across the heritabilities was 0.42, which suggests that nearly one fifth of the variance in the association between depressive symptoms and CAD was attributable to common genetic factors. In the Swedish population-based twin registry, only modest lifetime associations (around 30%) between major depression and CAD were observed. In women the genetic association was smaller but consistent throughout the life course, whereas in men the genetic association was stronger in younger age groups [101]. In a small selected male twin study from the Vietnam Era Twin Registry, carried out in people who were free of symptomatic CAD and major depressive disorder, current depressive symptoms (measured with the Beck Depression Inventory-II) were associated with IL-6 and CRP. Genetic modelling found a small and just significant genetic correlation between IL-6 and depressive symptoms $(r(G) = 0.22, \ p = 0.046)$ indicating that about 66% of the covariance between them can be explained by shared genetic influences [102].

The same candidate inflammatory genes that are contenders for the depression–CAD link may also be involved in the depression–diabetes link, if diabetes and CAD are considered as having similar biological origins and are along a related continuum of progressive metabolic dysfunction. In the field of type 2 diabetes, decades of intense research activity and linkage studies, and recently genome-wide association scans to identify candidate genes, have been moderately successful in identifying some, around 20, disease-susceptibility loci, although these mostly exert small effects on the risk of type 2 diabetes [96].

To date, little research has been conducted to explore directly the depression–diabetes link and what has been done seems to have had negative results. In a small male twin study, while depressive symptoms as measured by the Center for Epidemiologic Studies Scale were associated with metabolic risk factors (blood pressure, BMI, waist to hip ratio, serum triglycerides and fasting glucose), twin structural equation modelling indicated that the associations were attributable to environmental rather than genetic factors [103].

An area that has been neglected in recent years is the genetic basis of the dopamine reward systems. It has been suggested that this may be relevant to patterns of overeating and why satiety in some persons is higher than others. Reductions in dopamine $D_2$ receptor availability in the striatum have been demonstrated in people with obesity, and this has been likened to the deficiencies in the dopamine reward mechanisms in people with substance misuse and binge eating [104]. Binge eating traits seem to run in families and may be a mediator for obesity [105]. Obese individuals with a binge eating disorder are significantly more likely to have a family history of substance abuse than those in the general population, leading to the suggestion that compulsive disorders, such as drug addiction, gambling and obesity, reflect a 'reward deficiency syndrome' [106] that is thought to be due, in part, to a reduction in dopamine $D_2$ receptors.

In the last few years, there has been the development of new methodologies and guidelines in conducting gene-environment research. The availability of large data sets has led to increased power in both discovery of new candidate genes and replication studies. The emergence of genotyping technologies, such as single nucleotide polymorphisms, has opened up the opportunity for large scale study of genetic variants. The Human Genome Sequencing Project has increased understanding of patterns of sequence variation, such as copy number variation and low-frequency polymorphisms. It is now possible to undertake genome-wide surveys of common variant associations, and methodologies for assessing the combined genetic risk for common complex traits, such as depression and diabetes, are likely to be developed in the coming years. While it is likely that most genetic associations of depression and diabetes individually will continue to be of small to modest sizes, in the case of the depression–diabetes link any associations may reflect a more serious prognostic risk factor or subgroup, which may be of potential clinical importance.

## THE DIABETES–DEPRESSION LINK AND BIRTH WEIGHT

Since the emergence of the 'foetal origins' hypothesis of adult disease in the 1990s [107], which postulates that foetal undernutrition is independently associated with increased susceptibility to the development of CAD and related conditions in later life, there have been numerous studies testing this association. With regard to diabetes, a recent thorough systematic review found that in 23 populations an inverse association between birth weight and type 2 diabetes was observed, compared to positive associations in eight populations [108]. In a sensitivity analysis, in which studies that had strong positive associations were removed, the pooled age- and sex-adjusted odds ratio for type 2 diabetes was 0.75 (95% CI 0.70–0.81) per kilogram in the remaining 28 populations. The shape of the birth weight–type 2 diabetes association was strongly graded, particularly at birth weights of 3 kg or less.

The extent to which the foetal hypothesis applies to adult depression is less certain. It was first observed as a potential contributor to late-life depression, but since then the handful of studies have been not been convincing [109]. In the 1970 British Cohort Study, participants completed the 12-item General Health Questionnaire when they were aged 16 years, and at age 26 they completed the Malaise Inventory and a self-report history of depression. In women, having a birth weight of $\leq 3$ kg was associated with a 30% increased risk of being depressed at age 26 (OR = 1.3, 95% CI 1.0–1.5) compared with those who weighed > 3.5 kg. However, birth weight was not associated with self-report history of depression in adult life or with psychological distress at age 16. In men, only a lower birth weight, $\leq 2.5$ kg, was associated with a 60% increased risk of having psychological distress at age 16 and with reporting a history of depression at age 26 compared to those who weighed > 2.5 kg [110]. In the Southampton Women's Survey Study (n = 5830), there was no association between birth weight and depressive symptoms in adult life as measured on the 12-item General Health Questionnaire [111].

There is some evidence of programming of the HPA axis and the SNS in early life and this has been proposed as a mediating mechanism for a variety of stress-related disorders, as well as for cardiovascular and metabolic disorders [112].

The notion that poor foetal nutrition influences metabolic programming and mental health into adult life is a plausible one. The hypothesis that the intra-uterine environment influences the stress response phenotype is particularly attractive, as it provides a potentially unifying model for the depression–diabetes link. However, it remains at present unproven, at least in humans. The main methodological problem is that birth weight is a poor proxy marker of the foetal environmental. Another challenge for researchers is that there may be a curvilinear association between birth weight and type 2 diabetes (and possibly depression). Low birth weight, for whatever reason, such as food rationing or maternal depression [113], may lead to the body being programmed to overfeed. As mothers become more overweight with the epidemic of obesity and as the prevalence of type 2 diabetes increases, this will lead to a tendency to produce larger offspring, which is also associated with increased risk of type 2 diabetes [114]. Whether overweight babies also lead to increased risk for depression has yet to be determined. Few birth cohorts exist that have measured/are measuring detailed biological variables along the life course. As these are mostly in developed nations, their generalizability will be limited.

## THE DIABETES–DEPRESSION LINK AND EARLY CHILDHOOD ADVERSITY

Searching for clues for common etiological factors for depression and diabetes may be more fruitful in life course epidemiology. The life course perspective goes beyond conventional epidemiology by focusing on the 'long-term effects on chronic disease risk of physical and social exposures during gestation, childhood, adolescence, young adulthood and later adult life. It includes studies of the biological, behavioural and psychosocial pathways that operate across an individual's life course, as well as across generations, to influence the development of chronic diseases' [115]. Various designs exist which aim to measure the combination, accumulation and/or interactions of different environments and experiences throughout life that could potentially affect risk of CAD in adult life. This is a methodology which is still to emerge in its application to studying comorbidity, but potentially holds promise in unraveling causal or common pathways. A systematic review found consistent support for the detrimental impact of the accumulation of negative socioeconomic status across the life course on CAD risk [116], but this has not been shown for diabetes [108, 117, 118].

Educational attainment in childhood may be an important risk factor for depression–diabetes comorbidity, as was recently observed in a secondary analysis of the Baltimore Epidemiological Catchment Area Study. This is a population-based cohort study that began in 1981 and followed up for 23 years. Using a structured diagnostic interview and self-report of incident cases of diabetes, the investigators found that those who only completed high school had a greater association between depression and incident diabetes than those who went on to further education [119].

Life course epidemiology can help tease out the relative importance of early events compared to those in adult life and the role of biological markers for metabolic and cardiac disorders. In the Dunedin Multidisciplinary Health and Development Study, which is a birth cohort study currently followed up to age 32 years, the association between childhood maltreatment and adult inflammation was assessed taking into account multiple biological, psychological and social variables along the life course. Children who suffered maltreatment showed a significant and dose response increase by 80% in the risk for clinically relevant (concerning risk for CAD) CRP levels in adulthood, independent of the influence of co-occurring early life risks, such as birth weight, other stressors during adolescence and adulthood, adult anthropometry and health behaviours such as smoking [94, 95].

There are no studies to date that compare the risk factors for diabetes and depression over the life course in the same sample. The notion that in both depression and diabetes there is the accumulation of similar risk factors along the life course is appealingly plausible and has some face validity. As birth cohorts mature, such as the 1946 Medical Research Council Birth Cohorts and the Avon Longitudinal Study of Parents and Children, there will be more possibilities to explore how risk factors alter the health trajectories and have long-term effects on the diabetes–depression link.

## THE ROLE OF ANTIDEPRESSANTS

There is a potentially important role for antidepressants in helping to understand the pathogenesis of the depression–diabetes link. Antidepressants could have a positive effect either directly on the biological processes along the diabetes continuum or indirectly by improving mood and, therefore, health behaviours relating to diet and activity.

Based on mainly anecdotal evidence and a handful of randomized controlled trials, monoamine oxidase inhibitors and tricyclic anti-depressants are considered to have a hyperglycaemic effect, which is in keeping with their noradrenergic and/or appetitogenic effects, while selective serotonin reuptake inhibitors, such as fluoxetine and sertraline, are more likely to be anorectic, improve insulin sensitivity and reduce glucose levels, probably because the central serotoninergic pathways are important in the regulation of food intake and food preferences.

There is partial evidence that treatment of depression with anti-depressants does improve metabolic status, in particular insulin resistance [35–37], but also possibly glycaemic control [120] and weight loss [121]. It is, therefore, no surprise that one of the currently popular weight-reducing drugs in obesity, sibutramine, which is a serotonin and noradrenaline reuptake inhibitor, was originally developed as an antidepressant [122]. It is believed that its anorectic effect is mediated by the inhibition of the uptake of brain serotonin and noradrenaline.

To confuse the antidepressant story further are findings from the US Diabetes Prevention Program [123]. Around 5.7% of the sample self-reported to be taking antidepressants at baseline, and this was associated with a twofold to threefold increase in diabetes risk in those randomized to placebo and to the lifestyle intervention after adjusting for likely confounders. Among those randomized to the third group, metformin, antidepressant use was not associated with developing diabetes. In observational studies, including secondary analyses nested within randomized controlled trials, such as the Diabetes Prevention Program, the interpretation of the impact of antidepressant use on diabetes risk is multiple. Firstly, the assessment of the use of antidepressants is thwarted with biases, especially if self-reported. Secondly, antidepressant treatment is likely confounded by the severity of depression. Patients with more severe depression are more likely to be treated, but severity is also the best predictor for non-response. Thus, treated patients may not have a better depression outcome, especially in primary care systems where few receive guideline-level pharmacotherapy or increased intensity of antidepressant treatment based on persistent symptoms.

An alternative or additional mechanism by which antidepressants may have a positive effect on glucose metabolism is that they have an immunomodulating effect, observed mostly in animal models and cultured cells [124]. Clomipramine and imipramine have been shown to reduce the levels of pro-inflammatory cytokines TNF-$\alpha$, IL-1$\beta$ and IL-6 and to induce apoptosis of human lymphocytes [125], whereas escitalopram and citalopram have been found to increase the levels of anti-inflammatory cytokines, such as IL-10 [124]. There is also evidence that clomipramine and imipramine have a central anti-inflammatory effect on microglia cells, astrocytes and macrophages [126]. In a small randomized controlled trial, paroxetine attenuated interferon-alpha induced depression in humans with malignant melanoma [127].

## CONCLUSIONS

Recent research on the pathogenesis of the depression–diabetes link has identified numerous potential mechanisms, many of which are related to each other in terms of being on the same causal pathway. Thus, metabolic programming at genetic level and early nutrition (*in utero* and childhood), environmental stressors (childhood adversity and socioeconomic adversity in adulthood) and the obesogenic modern lifestyle individually and collectively induce overactivity of the HPA axis. Chronic functional hypercortisolaemia and chronic activation of the SNS appear to be linked to a constellation of pathophysiological processes, which include activation of the innate cell-mediated immune response, accumulation of visceral fat and insulin resistance, which ultimately progresses into type 2 diabetes. Depression is likely to play a role in several ways: as a coincidental consequence of the same environmental factors, namely environmental stressors, that influence glucose metabolism; as an independent factor that also influences nutrition and lifestyle behaviours; as a phenotype for a range of stress-related disorders which have a unifying overactivation of the HPA and inflammatory response to stress; and as a marker of severity of the underlying pathogenesis of diabetes. Overall, the evidence is pointing towards the depression–diabetes link having to some extent a common origin in which some individuals are more vulnerable (or are programmed) such that there is overactivation of those stress regulation pathways which contribute to metabolic dysregulation.

The evidence for these putative links is small, and the findings are not always consistent, but the literature is growing at a rapid pace, to the extent that opportunities for laboratory biomarkers as prognostic indicators of depression in type 2 diabetes could be at the bedside over the next decade. The importance of expanding new frontiers in the pharmacological treatment of both depression and diabetes, in particular considering whether antidepressants have anti-diabetes effects and the potential role of as yet undiscovered anti-inflammatory agents, cannot be understated, considering the prevalence of the depression–diabetes link and its poor prognosis.

## REFERENCES

1. Ismail, K., Sloggett, A., and De Stavola, B. (2000) Do common mental disorders increase cigarette consumption? Results from 5 waves of a population based panel cohort. *Am. J. Epidemiol.*, **152**, 651–657.
2. Sanchez-Villegas, A., Ara, I., Guillén-Grima, F. *et al.* (2008) Physical activity, sedentary index, and mental disorders in the SUN cohort study. *Med. Sci. Sports Exerc.*, **40**, 827–834.
3. Kivimäki, M., Lawlor, D.A., Singh-Manoux, A. *et al.* (2009) Common mental disorder and obesity: insight from four repeat measures over 19 years: prospective Whitehall II cohort study. *BMJ*, **339**, 3765.
4. Ciechanowski, P., Katon, W., and Russo, J. (2000) Depression and diabetes: impact of depressive symptoms on adherence, function, and costs. *Arch. Intern. Med.*, **160**, 3278–3285.
5. Egede, L., Ellis, C., and Grubaugh, A. (2009) The effect of depression on self-care behaviors and quality of care in a national sample of adults with diabetes. *Gen. Hosp. Psychiatry*, **31**, 422–427.
6. Katon, W., Von Korff, M., Ciechanowski, P. *et al.* (2004) Behavioral and clinical factors associated with depression among individuals with diabetes. *Diabetes Care*, **27**, 914–920.
7. Katon, W., Russo, J., Heckbert, S. *et al.* (2010) The relationship between changes in depression symptoms and changes in health risk behaviors in patients with diabetes. *Int. J. Geriatr. Psychiatry*, **25**, 466–475.
8. Golden, S.H., Lazo, M., Carnethon, M. *et al.* (2008) Examining a bidirectional association between depressive symptoms and diabetes. *JAMA*, **299**, 2751–2759.
9. Knol, M., Twisk, J., Beekman, A. *et al.* (2006) Depression as a risk factor for the onset of type 2 diabetes mellitus. A meta-analysis. *Diabetologia*, **49**, 837–845.
10. Mezuk, B., Eaton, W., Albrecht, S., and Golden, S.H. (2008) Depression and type 2 diabetes over the lifespan. *Diabetes Care*, **31**, 2383–2390.
11. Lustman, P., Anderson, R., Freedland, K. *et al.* (2000) Depression and poor glycaemic control. A meta-analytic review of the literature. *Diabetes Care*, **23**, 934–942.
12. Kivimäki, M., Tabak, A., Batty, G. *et al.* (2009) Hyperglycemia, type 2 diabetes, and depressive symptoms: the British Whitehall II study. *Diabetes Care*, **32**, 1870–1872.
13. Katon, W., Rutter, C., Simon, G. *et al.* (2005) The association of comorbid depression with mortality in patients with type 2 diabetes. *Diabetes Care*, **28**, 2668–2672.

14. Nakahara, R., Yoshiuchi, K., Kumano, H. *et al.* (2006) Prospective study on influence of psychosocial factors on glycemic control in Japanese patients with type 2 diabetes. *Psychosomatics*, **47**, 240–246.

15. Ismail, K., Winkley, K., Stahl, D. *et al.* (2007) A cohort study of people with diabetes and their first foot ulcer: the role of depression on mortality. *Diabetes Care*, **30**, 1473–1479.

16. Fisher, L., Mullan, J., Arean, P. *et al.* (2010) Diabetes distress and not clinical depression or depressive symptoms is associated with glycemic control in both cross-sectional and longitudinal analyses. *Diabetes Care*, **33**, 23–28.

17. Aikens, J.E., Perkins, D.W., Lipton, B., and Piette, J.D. (2009) Longitudinal analysis of depressive symptoms and glycemic control in type 2 diabetes. *Diabetes Care*, **32**, 1177–1181.

18. Richardson, L.K., Egede, L.E., Mueller, M. *et al.* (2008) Longitudinal effects of depression on glycemic control in veterans with type 2 diabetes. *Gen. Hosp. Psychiatry*, **30**, 509–514.

19. Petrak, F. and Herpertz, S. (2009) Treatment of depression in diabetes – an update. *Curr. Opin. Psychiatry*, **22**, 211–217.

20. Pickup, J. (2004) Inflammation and activated innate immunity in the pathogenesis of type 2 diabetes. *Diabetes Care*, **27**, 813–823.

21. Carney, R., Rich, M., Freedland, K. *et al.* (1988) Major depressive disorder predicts cardiac events in patients with coronary artery disease. *Psychosom. Med.*, **50**, 627–633.

22. Frasure-Smith, N., Lesperance, F., and Talajic, M. (1993) Depression following myocardial infarction. Impact on 6-month survival. *JAMA*, **270**, 1819–1825.

23. Nicholson, A., Kuper, H., and Hemingway, H. (2006) Depression as an aetiologic and prognostic factor in coronary heart disease: a meta-analysis of 6362 events among 146 538 participants in 54 observational studies. *Eur. Heart J.*, **27**, 2763–2774.

24. Glassman, A.H., Bigger, J.T. Jr., and Gaffney, M. (2009) Psychiatric characteristics associated with long-term mortality among 361 patients having an acute coronary syndrome and major depression: seven-year follow-up of SADHART participants. *Arch. Gen. Psychiatry*, **66**, 1022–1029.

25. Penninx, B., Beekman, A., Honig, A. *et al.* (2001) Depression and cardiac mortality: results from a community-based longitudinal study. *Arch. Gen. Psychiatry*, **58**, 221–227.

26. Glassman, A.H., O'Connor, C.M., Califf, R.M. *et al.* (2002) Sertraline treatment of major depression in patients with acute MI or unstable angina. *JAMA*, **288**, 701–709.

27. Writing Committee for the ENRICHD Investigators (2003) Effects of treating depression and low perceived social support on clinical events after myocardial infarction: the Enhancing Recovery in Coronary Heart Disease Patients (ENRICHD) randomized trial. *JAMA*, **289**, 3106–3116.

28. Li, L. and Hölscher, C. (2007) Common pathological processes in Alzheimer's disease and type 2 diabetes: a review. *Brain Res. Rev.*, **56**, 384–402.

29. Lawlor, D.A., Smith, G.D., and Ebrahim, S. (2003) Association of insulin resistance with depression: cross sectional findings from the British Women's Heart and Health study. *BMJ*, **327**, 1383–1384.

30. Timonen, M., Laakso, M., Jokelainen, J. *et al.* (2005) Insulin resistance and depression: cross sectional study. *BMJ*, **330**, 17–18.

31. Adriaanse, M., Dekker, J., Nijpels, G. *et al.* (2006) Associations between depressive symptoms and insulin resistance: the Hoorn study. *Diabetologia*, **49**, 2874–2877.

32. Pan, A., Ye, X., Franco, O.H. *et al.* (2008) Insulin resistance and depressive symptoms in middle-aged and elderly Chinese: findings from the Nutrition and Health of Aging Population in China study. *J. Affect. Disord.*, **109**, 75–82.

33. Timonen, M., Salmenkaita, I., Jokelainen, J. *et al.* (2007) Insulin resistance and depressive symptoms in young adult males: findings from Finnish military conscripts. *Psychosom. Med.*, **69**, 723–728.

34. Timonen, M., Rajala, U., Jokelainen, J. *et al.* (2006) Depressive symptoms and insulin resistance in young adult males: results from the Northern Finland 1966 Birth Cohort. *Mol. Psychiatry*, **11**, 929–933.

35. Okamura, F., Tashiro, A., Utumi, A. *et al.* (2000) Insulin resistance in patients with depression and its changes during the clinical course of depression: minimal model analysis. *Metabolism*, **49**, 1255–1260.

36. Weber-Hamann, B., Gilles, M., Lederbogen, F. *et al.* (2006) Improved insulin sensitivity in 80 nondiabetic patients with MDD after clinical remission in a double-blind, randomized trial of amitriptyline and paroxetine. *J. Clin. Psychiatry*, **67**, 1856–1861.

37. Kauffman, R.P., Castracane, V.D., White, D.L. *et al.* (2005) Impact of the selective serotonin reuptake inhibitor citalopram on insulin sensitivity, leptin and basal cortisol secretion in depressed and non-depressed euglycemic women of reproductive age. *Gynecol. Endocrinol.*, **21**, 129–137.

38. Everson-Rose, S.A., Meyer, P.M., Powell, L.H. *et al.* (2004) Depressive symptoms, insulin resistance, and risk of diabetes in women at midlife. *Diabetes Care*, **27**, 2856–2862.

39. Lawlor, D., Yoav Ben-Shlomo, Y., Ebrahim, S. *et al.* (2005) Insulin resistance and depressive symptoms in middle aged men: findings from the Caerphilly prospective cohort study. *BMJ*, **330**, 705–706.

40. Brotman, D., Golden, S., and Wittstein, I. (2007) The cardiovascular toll of stress. *Lancet*, **370**, 1089–1100.

41. Anagnostis, P., Athyros, V.G., Tziomalos, K. *et al.* (2009) The pathogenetic role of cortisol in the metabolic syndrome: a hypothesis. *J. Clin. Endocrinol. Metab.*, **94**, 2692–2701.

42. Bjorntorp, P. (1991) Visceral fat accumulation: the missing link between psychosocial factors and cardiovascular disease? *J. Intern. Med.*, **230**, 195–201.

43. Bjorntorp, P. (1993) Visceral obesity: a 'civilisation syndrome'. *Obes. Res.*, **1**, 206–222.

44. Pariante, C.M. and Miller, A.H. (2001) Glucocorticoid receptors in major depression: relevance to pathophysiology and treatment. *Biol. Psychiatry*, **49**, 391–404.

45. Burke, H., Davis, M., Otte, C., and Mohr, D. (2005) Depression and cortisol responses to psychological stress: a meta-analysis. *Psychoneuroendocrinology*, **30**, 846–856.

46. Shea, A., Walsh, C., MacMillan, H., and Steiner, M. (2005) Child maltreatment and HPA axis dysregulation: relationship to major depressive disorder and post traumatic stress disorder in females. *Psychoneuroendocrinology*, **30**, 162–178.

47. Belmaker, R.H. and Agam, G. (2008) Major depressive disorder. *N. Engl. J. Med.*, **358**, 55–68.

48. Rush, A., Giles, D., Schlesser, M. *et al.* (1996) The dexamethasone suppression test in patients with mood disorders. *J. Clin. Psychiatry*, **57**, 470–484.

49. Vreeburg, S.A., Hoogendijk, W.J.G., van Pelt, J. *et al.* (2009) Major depressive disorder and hypothalamic-pituitary-adrenal axis activity: results from a large cohort study. *Arch. Gen. Psychiatry*, **66**, 617–626.

50. Fountoulakis, K., Gonda, X., Rihmer, Z. *et al.* (2008) Revisiting the dexamethasone suppression test in unipolar major depression: an exploratory study. *Ann. Gen. Psychiatry*, **7**, 22.

51. Otte, C., Marmar, C.R., Pipkin, S.S. *et al.* (2004) Depression and 24-hour urinary cortisol in medical outpatients with coronary heart disease: the Heart and Soul study. *Biol. Psychiatry*, **56**, 241–247.

52. Steptoe, A., O'Donnell, K., Badrick, E. *et al.* (2008) Neuroendocrine and inflammatory factors associated with positive affect in healthy men and women: the Whitehall II study. *Am. J. Epidemiol.*, **167**, 96–102.

53. Larsson, C., Gullberg, B., Rastam, L., and Lindblad, U. (2009) Salivary cortisol differs with age and sex and shows inverse associations with WHR in Swedish women: a cross-sectional study. *BMC Endocr. Disord.*, **9**, 16.

54. Bartels, M., Van den Berg, M., Sluyter, F. *et al.* (2003) Heritability of cortisol levels: review and simultaneous analysis of twin studies. *Psychoneuroendocrinology*, **28**, 121–137.

55. Otte, C., Wüst, S., Zhao, S. *et al.* (2009) Glucocorticoid receptor gene and depression in patients with coronary heart disease: the Heart and Soul study – 2009 Curt Richter award winner. *Psychoneuroendocrinology*, **34**, 1574–1581.

56. Goodyer, I.M., Bacon, A., Ban, M. *et al.* (2009) Serotonin transporter genotype, morning cortisol and subsequent depression in adolescents. *Br. J. Psychiatry*, **195**, 39–45.

57. Matta, S.G., Fu, Y., Valentine, J.D., and Sharp, B.M. (1998) Response of the hypothalamo-pituitary-adrenal axis to nicotine. *Psychoneuroendocrinology*, **23**, 103–113.

58. de Kloet, C., Vermetten, E., Geuze, E. *et al.* (2006) Assessment of HPA-axis function in posttraumatic stress disorder: pharmacological and non-pharmacological challenge tests, a review. *J. Psychiatr. Res.*, **40**, 550–567.

59. Nater, U., Maloney, E., Boneva, R. *et al.* (2008) Attenuated morning salivary cortisol concentrations in a population-based study of persons with chronic fatigue syndrome and well controls. *J. Clin. Endocrinol. Metab.*, **93**, 703–709.

60. Mondelli, V., Dazzan, P., Hepgul, N. *et al.* (2010) Abnormal cortisol levels during the day and cortisol awakening response in first-episode psychosis: the role of stress and of antipsychotic treatment. *Schizophr. Res.*, **116**, 234–242.

61. Ismail, K., Murray, R., Wheeler, M., and O'Keane, V. (1998) The dexamethasone suppression test in schizophrenia. *Psychol Med.*, **28**, 311–317.

62. Heim, C., Newport, D.J., Heit, S. *et al.* (2000) Pituitary-adrenal and autonomic responses to stress in women after sexual and physical abuse in childhood. *JAMA*, **284**, 592–597.

63. Heim, C., Nater, U.M., Maloney, E. *et al.* (2009) Childhood trauma and risk for chronic fatigue syndrome: association with neuroendocrine dysfunction. *Arch. Gen. Psychiatry*, **66**, 72–80.

64. Harris, T., Borsanyi, S., Messari, S. *et al.* (2000) Morning cortisol as a risk factor for subsequent major depressive disorder in adult women. *Br. J. Psychiatry*, **177**, 505–510.

65. Goodyer, I., Tamplin, A., Herbert, J., and Altham, P. (2000) Recent life events, cortisol, dehydroepiandrosterone and the onset of major depression in high-risk adolescents. *Br. J. Psychiatry*, **177**, 499–504.

66. Zhao, W.-Q. and Townsend, M. (2009) Insulin resistance and amyloidogenesis as common molecular foundation for type 2 diabetes and Alzheimer's disease. *BBA-Mol. Basis Dis.*, **1792**, 482–496.

67. Vogelzangs, N., Suthers, K., Ferrucci, L. *et al.* (2007) Hypercortisolemic depression is associated with the metabolic syndrome in late-life. *Psychoneuroendocrinology*, **32**, 151–159.

68. Hudson, J.I., Hudson, M.S., Rothschild, A.J. *et al.* (1984) Abnormal results of dexamethasone suppression tests in nondepressed patients with diabetes mellitus. *Arch. Gen. Psychiatry*, **41**, 1086–1089.

69. Carney, R.M., Freedland, K.E., and Veith, R.C. (2005) Depression, the autonomic nervous system, and coronary heart disease. *Psychosom. Med.*, **67**, S29–S33.

70. Rottenberg, J. (2007) Cardiac vagal control in depression: a critical analysis. *Biol. Psychol.*, **74**, 200–211.

71. Licht, C.M.M., de Geus, E.J.C., Zitman, F.G. *et al.* (2008) Association between major depressive disorder and heart rate variability in the Netherlands Study of Depression and Anxiety (NESDA). *Arch. Gen. Psychiatry*, **65**, 1358–1367.

72. Ohira, T., Roux, A.V.D., Prineas, R.J. *et al.* (2008) Associations of psychosocial factors with heart rate and its short-term variability: Multiethnic Study of Atherosclerosis. *Psychosom. Med.*, **70**, 141–146.

73. Carney, R.M., Blumenthal, J.A., Stein, P.K. *et al.* (2001) Depression, heart rate variability, and acute myocardial infarction. *Circulation*, **104**, 2024–2028.

74. Gehi, A., Mangano, D., Pipkin, S. *et al.* (2005) Depression and heart rate variability in patients with stable coronary heart disease: findings from the Heart and Soul study. *Arch. Gen. Psychiatry*, **62**, 661–666.

75. Vinik, A.I., Maser, R.E., Mitchell, B.D., and Freeman, R. (2003) Diabetic autonomic neuropathy. *Diabetes Care*, **26**, 1553–1579.

76. Talley, S.J., Bytzer, P., Hammer, J. *et al.* (2001) Psychological distress is linked to gastrointestinal symptoms in diabetes mellitus. *Am. J. Gastroenterol.*, **96**, 1033–1038.

77. Ludman, E.J., Katon, W., Russo, J. *et al.* (2004) Depression and diabetes symptom burden. *Gen. Hosp. Psychiatry*, **26**, 430–436.

78. Smith, R. (1991) The macrophage theory of depression. *Med. Hypotheses*, **36**, 178.

79. Pickup, J. and Crook, M. (1998) Is type II diabetes a disease of the innate immune system? *Diabetologia*, **41**, 1241–1248.

80. Fernández-Real, J.M. and Pickup, J.C. (2008) Innate immunity, insulin resistance and type 2 diabetes. *Trends Endocrinol. Metab.*, **19**, 10–16.

81. Pradhan, A.D., Manson, J.E., Rifai, N. *et al.* (2001) C-reactive protein, interleukin 6, and risk of developing type 2 diabetes mellitus. *JAMA*, **286**, 327–334.

82. Cesari, M., Penninx, B.W.J.H., Newman, A.B. *et al.* (2003) Inflammatory markers and onset of cardiovascular events: results from the Health ABC study. *Circulation*, **108**, 2317–2322.

83. Li, S., Shin, H.J., Ding, E.L., and van Dam, R.M. (2009) Adiponectin levels and risk of type 2 diabetes: a systematic review and meta-analysis. *JAMA*, **302**, 179–188.

84. Pickup, J. and Mattock, M. (2003) Activation of the innate immune system as a predictor of cardiovascular mortality in type 2 diabetes mellitus. *Diabet. Med.*, **20**, 723–726.

85. Larsen, C.M., Faulenbach, M., Vaag, A. *et al.* (2007) Interleukin-1-receptor antagonist in type 2 diabetes mellitus. *N. Engl. J. Med.*, **356**, 1517–1526.

86. Larsen, C.M., Faulenbach, M., Vaag, A. *et al.* (2009) Sustained effects of interleukin-1 receptor antagonist treatment in type 2 diabetes. *Diabetes Care*, **32**, 1663–1668.

87. Herder, C., Peltonen, M., Koenig, W. *et al.* (2006) Systemic immune mediators and lifestyle changes in the prevention of type 2 diabetes. *Diabetes*, **55**, 2340–2346.

88. Howren, M.B., Lamkin, D.M., and Suls, J. (2009) Associations of depression with c-reactive protein, IL-1, and IL-6: a meta-analysis. *Psychosom. Med.*, **71**, 171–186.

89. Ferketich, A.K., Ferguson, J.P., and Binkley, P.F. (2005) Depressive symptoms and inflammation among heart failure patients. *Am. Heart J.*, **150**, 132–136.

90. Danese, A., Pariante, C.M., Caspi, A. *et al.* (2007) Childhood maltreatment predicts adult inflammation in a life-course study. *Proc. Natl. Acad. Sci. USA*, **104**, 1319–1324.

91. Fuligni, A.J., Telzer, E.H., Bower, J. *et al.* (2009) A preliminary study of daily interpersonal stress and C-reactive protein levels among adolescents from Latin American and European backgrounds. *Psychosom. Med.*, **71**, 329–333.

92. Davidson, K.W., Schwartz, J.E., Kirkland, S.A. *et al.* (2009) Relation of inflammation to depression and incident coronary heart disease (from the Canadian Nova Scotia Health Survey [NSHS95] prospective population study). *Am. J. Cardiol.*, **103**, 755–761.

93. Vaccarino, V., Johnson, B., Sheps, D. *et al.* (2007) Depression, inflammation, and incident cardiovascular disease in women with suspected coronary ischemia: the National Heart, Lung, and Blood Institute-sponsored study. *J. Am. Coll. Cardiol.*, **50**, 2044–2050.

94. Golden, S.H., Lee, H.B., Schreiner, P.J. *et al.* (2007) Depression and type 2 diabetes mellitus: the Multiethnic Study of Atherosclerosis. *Psychosom. Med.*, **69**, 529–536.

95. Maes, M., Yirmyia, R., Noraberg, J. *et al.* (2009) The inflammatory & neurodegenerative (I & ND) hypothesis of depression: leads for future research and new drug developments in depression. *Metab. Brain Dis.*, **24**, 27–53.

96. McCarthy, M. and Eleftheria Zeggini, E. (2009) Genome-wide association studies in type 2 diabetes. *Curr. Diabetes Rep.*, **9**, 164–171.

97. Sullivan, P.F., Neale, M.C., and Kendler, K.S. (2000) Genetic epidemiology of major depression: review and meta-analysis. *Am. J. Psychiatry*, **157**, 1552–1562.

98. McCaffery, J.M., Frasure-Smith, N., Dube, M.-P. *et al.* (2006) Common genetic vulnerability to depressive symptoms and coronary artery disease: a review and development of candidate genes related to inflammation and serotonin. *Psychosom. Med.*, **68**, 187–200.

99. Risch, N., Herrell, R., Lehner, T. *et al.* (2009) Interaction between the serotonin transporter gene (5-HTTLPR), stressful life events, and risk of depression: a meta-analysis. *JAMA*, **301**, 2462–2471.

100. Otte, C., McCaffery, J., Ali, S., and Whooley, M.A. (2007) Association of a serotonin transporter polymorphism (5-HTTLPR) with depression, perceived stress, and norepinephrine in patients with coronary disease: the Heart and Soul study. *Am. J. Psychiatry*, **164**, 1379–1384.

101. Kendler, K.S., Gardner, C.O., Fiske, A., and Gatz, M. (2009) Major depression and coronary artery disease in the Swedish twin registry: phenotypic, genetic, and environmental sources of comorbidity. *Arch. Gen. Psychiatry*, **66**, 857–863.

102. Su, S., Miller, A.H., Snieder, H. *et al.* (2009) Common genetic contributions to depressive symptoms and inflammatory markers in middle-aged men: the Twins Heart Study. *Psychosom. Med.*, **71**, 152–158.

103. McCaffery, J.M., Niaura, R., Todaro, J.F. *et al.* (2003) Depressive symptoms and metabolic risk in adult male twins enrolled in the National Heart, Lung, and Blood Institute Twin Study. *Psychosom. Med.*, **65**, 490–497.

104. Wang, G.-J., Volkow, N., Logan, J. *et al.* (2001) Brain dopamine and obesity. *Lancet*, **357**, 354–357.

105. Hudson, J.I., Lalonde, J.K., Berry, J.M. *et al.* (2006) Binge-eating disorder as a distinct familial phenotype in obese individuals. *Arch. Gen. Psychiatry*, **63**, 313–319.

106. Yanovski, S., Nelson, J., Dubbert, B., and Spitzer, R. (1993) Association of binge eating disorder and psychiatric comorbidity in obese subjects. *Am. J. Psychiatry*, **150**, 1472–1479.

107. Barker, D. (1995) Foetal origins of coronary heart disease. *BMJ*, **311**, 171–174.

108. Whincup, P.H., Kaye, S.J., Owen, C.G. *et al.* (2008) Birth weight and risk of type 2 diabetes: a systematic review. *JAMA*, **300**, 2886–2897.

109. Thompson, S., Auslander, W., and White, N. (2001) Comparison of single-mother and two-parent families on metabolic control of children with diabetes. *Diabetes Care*, **24**, 234–238.

110. Gale, C. and Martyn, C. (2004) Birth weight and later risk of depression in a national birth cohort. *Br. J. Psychiatry*, **184**, 28–33.

111. Inskip, H.M., Dunn, N., Godfrey, K.M. *et al.* (2008) Is birth weight associated with risk of depressive symptoms in young women? Evidence from the Southampton Women's survey. *Am. J. Epidemiol.*, **167**, 164–168.

112. Kajantie, E., Eriksson, J., Osmond, C. *et al.* (2004) Size at birth, the metabolic syndrome and 24-h salivary cortisol profile. *Clin. Endocrinol.*, **60**, 201–207.

113. Yonkers, K.A., Wisner, K.L., Stewart, D.E. *et al.* (2009) The management of depression during pregnancy: a report from the American Psychiatric Association and the American College of Obstetricians and Gynecologists. *Gen. Hosp. Psychiatry*, **31**, 403–413.

114. Kerényi, Z., Tamás, G., Kivimäki, M. *et al.* (2009) Maternal glycemia and risk of large-for-gestational-age babies in a population-based screening. *Diabetes Care*, **32**, 2200–2205.

115. Ben-Shlomo, Y. and Kuh, D. (2002) A life course approach to chronic disease epidemiology: conceptual models, empirical challenges and interdisciplinary perspectives. *Int. J. Epidemiol.*, **31**, 285–293.

116. Pollitt, R., Rose, K., and Kaufman, J. (2005) Evaluating the evidence for models of life course socioeconomic factors and cardiovascular outcomes: a systematic review. *BMC Public Health*, **5**, 7.

117. Andersen, A.F., Carson, C., Watt, H.C. *et al.* (2008) Life-course socioeconomic position, area deprivation and type 2 diabetes: findings from the British Women's Heart and Health Study. *Diabet. Med.*, **25**, 1462–1468.

118. Agardh, E., Ahlbom, A., Andersson, T. *et al.* (2007) Socio-economic position at three points in life in association with type 2 diabetes and

impaired glucose tolerance in middle-aged Swedish men and women. *Int. J. Epidemiol.*, **36**, 84–92.

119. Mezuk, B., Eaton, W.W., Golden, S.H., and Ding, Y. (2008) The influence of educational attainment on depression and risk of type 2 diabetes. *Am. J. Public Health*, **98**, 1480–1485.

120. Lustman, P., Clouse, R., Nix, B. *et al.* (2006) Sertraline for prevention of depression recurrence in diabetes mellitus. A randomized, double-blind, placebo-controlled trial. *Arch. Gen. Psychiatry*, **63**, 521–529.

121. Lustman, P.J., Williams, M.M., Sayuk, G.S. *et al.* (2007) Factors influencing glycemic control in type 2 diabetes during acute- and maintenance-phase treatment of major depressive disorder with bupropion. *Diabetes Care*, **30**, 459–466.

122. Arterburn, D.E., Crane, P.K., and Veenstra, D.L. (2004) The efficacy and safety of sibutramine for weight loss: a systematic review. *Arch. Intern. Med.*, **164**, 994–1003.

123. Rubin, R.R., Ma, Y., Marrero, D.G. *et al.* (2008) Elevated depression symptoms, antidepressant medicine use, and risk of developing diabetes during the Diabetes Prevention Program. *Diabetes Care*, **31**, 420–426.

124. Maes, M., Song, C., Lin, A. *et al.* (1999) Negative immunoregulatory effects of antidepressants: inhibition of interferon-gamma and stimulation of interleukin-10 secretion. *Neuropsychopharmacology*, **20**, 370–379.

125. Xia, Z., DePierre, J., and Nassberger, L. (1996) Tricyclic antidepressants inhibit IL-6, IL-1beta and TNF-alpha release in human blood monocytes and IL-2 and interferon-gamma in T cells. *Immunopharmacology*, **34**, 27–37.

126. Hwang, J., Zheng, L.T., Ock, J. *et al.* (2008) Inhibition of glial inflammatory activation and neurotoxicity by tricyclic antidepressants. *Neuropharmacology*, **55**, 826–834.

127. Musselman, D.L., Lawson, D.H., Gumnick, J.F. *et al.* (2001) Paroxetine for the prevention of depression induced by high-dose interferon alfa. *N. Engl. J. Med.*, **344**, 961–966.

# CHAPTER 3

# Medical Costs of Depression and Diabetes

**Leonard E. Egede**

*Department of Medicine, Center for Health Disparities Research, Medical University of South Carolina; and Center for Disease Prevention and Health Interventions for Diverse Populations, Ralph H. Johnson VA Medical Center, Charleston, SC, USA*

Diabetes mellitus is a chronic debilitating disease, with prevalence estimates that are approaching epidemic proportions worldwide. Estimates from the fourth edition of the International Diabetes Federation (IDF) Diabetes Atlas, published in 2009, show that 285 million people worldwide, or 6.6% of the world population, aged 20–79 would have diabetes in 2010 [1]. This number is expected to increase by 50% by 2030, when approximately 438 million people, or 7.8% of the adult population, are projected to have diabetes worldwide [1]. Diabetes is more prevalent among middle aged adults (ages 40–59 years), women and those who reside in urban areas [1].

Diabetes is expected to account for four million deaths among those aged 20–79 years globally in 2010 [1]. This will account for 6.8% of all-cause global mortality. The highest mortality rates are expected to occur in countries with large populations, such as India, China, the United States and the Russian Federation [1]. Current estimates show that diabetes mortality is higher in women compared to men, with diabetes accounting for a quarter of deaths in women in some populations [1].

*Depression and Diabetes* Edited by Wayne Katon, Mario Maj and Norman Sartorius
© 2010 John Wiley & Sons, Ltd

In the United States, 23.6 million people, or 7.8% of the population, had diabetes in 2007 [2]. Diabetes is more prevalent in ethnic minorities (Hispanic, African Americans and native Americans) [2]. It was the seventh leading cause of death in 2006 and the leading cause of blindness, kidney failure and non-traumatic lower limb amputations [2]. Adults with diabetes have twofold to fourfold increased deaths from heart disease and twofold to fourfold increased risk of stroke compared to adults without diabetes [2]. Thus, diabetes is a highly prevalent disease that is associated with significant morbidity and mortality worldwide.

Just like diabetes, depression is highly prevalent worldwide and associated with significant morbidity and mortality. Approximately 340 million people worldwide suffer from depression at any given time, including 18 million in the United States [3]. Based on estimates from the World Health Organization (WHO), depression is responsible for the greatest proportion of burden associated with non-fatal health outcomes and accounts for approximately 12% total years lived with disability [4]. In 2000, it was estimated that depressive disorders were higher in women (4930 per 100 000) than men (3199 per 100 000) and that globally depressive disorders were the fourth leading cause of disease burden in women and the seventh leading cause in men [5].

Recent studies have reported that the lifetime prevalence of a major depressive disorder in the United States was 16.2% [6], whereas the lifetime prevalence in Europe was 14% [7]. A third study designed to examine the prevalence of mood disorders in 14 countries in the Americas, Europe, Middle East, Africa and Asia found that the 12-month prevalence of mood disorders was 0.8% in Nigeria, 3.15 in Japan, 6.6% in Lebanon, 6.8% in Columbia, 6.9% in the Netherlands, 8.5% in France, 9.1% in the Ukraine and 9.6% in the United States [8]. However, estimates from international studies need to be interpreted with caution because of the absence of reliability data on diagnostic instruments for depression in several countries.

Studies show that depression is a major cause of morbidity, mortality and disability [9] and is associated with workplace absenteeism, diminished or lost work productivity and increased use of healthcare resources [10]. Finally, major depression is the second leading cause of disability-adjusted life years (DALYs) lost in women and the tenth leading cause of DALYs in men [9].

Multiple large epidemiological studies have established that depression is prevalent among adults with diabetes [11, 12]. In a large meta-analysis conducted by Anderson *et al.* [13], the prevalence of major depression in people with diabetes was 11% and the prevalence of clinically relevant depression was 31%. However, worldwide estimates of depression prevalence among individuals with diabetes appear to vary by diabetes type and among developed and developing nations. The World Mental Health Survey was conducted to estimate the 12-month prevalence rate of mood, anxiety and alcohol-use disorder among community samples of adults across 17 countries in Europe, the Americas, the Middle East, Africa, Asia and the South Pacific [14]. The risk of mood and anxiety disorders was higher among individuals with diabetes relative to those without. The odds ratio for depression was 1.38 (95% CI 1.14–1.66) after adjusting for age and gender.

In the United States, Li *et al.* [15] estimated the age-adjusted rates of depression in a nationally representative survey of adults aged 18 and older in 2006 and found that the age-adjusted rate of depression was 8.3% (95% CI 7.3–9.3), ranging from a low of 2.0% to a high of 28.8% among the 50 states. The authors conducted a second study using the same nationally representative survey in 2006 to estimate the prevalence of undiagnosed depression among individuals with diabetes [16]. In this second study, the adjusted and unadjusted prevalence of undiagnosed depression were 8.75 and 9.2%, respectively [16]. Elevated depressive symptoms have also been reported in African Americans residing in rural counties in Georgia [17] and urban primary clinics in East Baltimore, Maryland [18]. In a binational study (USA and Mexico) of more than 300 patients, Mier *et al.* [19] found that the rate of depression among Hispanic patients with diabetes was 39% in south Texas and 40.5% in north eastern Mexico.

Estimates of depression among individuals with diabetes from international studies are fairly consistent and show that depression is prevalent among adults with diabetes. In a study conducted in rural Bangladesh, Asghar *et al.* [20] found that 29% of men and 31% of women with newly diagnosed diabetes had depressive symptoms. In a study conducted in Greece, Sotiropoulos *et al.* [21] found that 33% of Greek adults with type 2 diabetes had symptoms of depression. A study conducted in rural Pakistan by Zahid *et al.* [22] found a depression prevalence of 15% among patients with diabetes. A study in Bahrain [23] found higher rates of moderate to severe depression in patients with type 2 diabetes. Among the international studies, the highest rate of depression in adults with diabetes was reported in Iran. In that study, approximately 72% of Iranian patients with diabetes had depression [24].

Ali *et al.* [25] performed a systematic review that included international studies to estimate the prevalence of clinically-relevant depression in adults with type 2 diabetes and found that the prevalence of depression was 17.6% among patients with type 2 diabetes compared to 9.8% among those without diabetes.

## MEDICAL COSTS OF DIABETES AND OF DEPRESSION

Diabetes is associated with increased healthcare use and cost. Global estimates of expenditure to treat and prevent diabetes and its complications are expected to reach (US)$376 billion in 2010 [1]. By 2030 this number is projected to exceed $490 billion. On average, it is estimated that $708 will be spent per adult with diabetes in 2010 [1].

The cost of diabetes selectively impacts middle aged and older adults. More than 75% of the global expenditure for diabetes will be made in adults between the ages of 50 and 80 years [1]. Expenditures for diabetes are also higher in developed and affluent countries compared to less developed countries, even though 70% of the world's population with diabetes lives in less developed countries. Current estimates show that 80% of total global expenditure for diabetes is made in the world's richest countries, where less than 30% of the world's population with diabetes lives, indicating substantial inequity in available resources for treating and preventing the complications of diabetes.

In the United States, cost estimates for diabetes in 2007 showed that total cost was $174 billion, of which $116 billion was due to direct medical cost and $58 billion was due to indirect costs, including disability, work loss and premature mortality [2]. Average medical expenditure in 2007 was 2.3 times higher for individuals with diagnosed diabetes compared to those without diabetes [2].

Depressive disorders impose substantial economic costs globally. One of the first major cost studies for depression in the United States used data from 1990 and showed that the annual total cost of depressive disorders was $43.7 billion [26]. Approximately 28% of the total cost in 1990 ($12.4 billion) was due to direct medical costs, whereas 17% ($7.5 billion) was due to mortality from suicide and 55% ($23.8 billion) was due to morbidity costs (indirect costs) associated with depression in the work place [26]. In another study, Druss *et al.* [27] found that major depression increased total healthcare costs per individual by $2907 and depressive symptoms increased total cost per individual by $1576. They also examined the healthcare cost of depressive illness in a major United States corporation and found that employees treated for depression incurred $5415 annual per capita costs, which were significantly higher than costs for hypertension, and similar to costs for diabetes and heart disease [28].

In another study, Druss *et al.* [29] compared the national economic burden of five chronic conditions in the United States based on 1996 data and found that total healthcare costs of individuals with depressive and manic-depressive disorders were $66.4 billion, which was higher than the total costs of heart disease, diabetes and asthma. Unutzer *et al.* [30] examined the association between depression and 12-month healthcare costs in 14 902 medically ill participants in a fee for service programme and found that depressed individuals had significantly higher total costs ($20 046 vs $11 956). The higher cost was consistent across almost every cost category examined, including home healthcare, skilled nursing facility, outpatient non-mental healthcare, inpatient non-mental healthcare, physician services and durable medical equipment costs. Consistent with the findings from United States studies, studies conducted in Taiwan [31] and China [32] also found that depression was associated with significant increases in healthcare costs in those countries.

Overall, the results of these studies indicate that the economic burden of depression both to the individual and to society is tremendous and is comparable to the economic burden of diabetes.

## IMPACT OF COEXISTING DEPRESSION AND DIABETES ON DISABILITY, PRODUCTIVITY AND QUALITY OF LIFE

Several studies have shown that comorbid depression is associated with decreased function and increased odds of lost productivity in people with diabetes. In the Hispanic Established Populations for

Epidemiologic Studies of the Elderly (EPESE) survey, the coexistence of diabetes and depression was associated with increased risk of disability among older Mexican Americans [33]. In that study, patients with diabetes and coexisting depression had 4.1-fold increased odds of disability, while those with diabetes alone and depression alone had 1.7-fold and 1.3-fold increased odds of disability, respectively. In another study, data on 30 022 adults from a representative sample of the United States population was analysed to determine the effect of depression on functional disability in adults with diabetes [34]. In that study, the odds of functional disability were 3.00 (95% CI 2.62–3.42) for adults with major depression, 2.42 (95% CI 2.10–2.79) for those with diabetes and 7.15 (95% CI 4.53–11.28) for those with both diabetes and depression. Another study assessed the effect of major depression on lost productivity in adults with diabetes [35]: individuals with diabetes and coexisting depression missed more days from work, spent more days in bed due to disability and were more likely to miss more than seven days of work in any given year.

In a study of 3010 Australian adults, the coexistence of diabetes and depression was associated with significantly lower physical and mental health component scores of the Short Form-36 (SF-36) scale compared to those with either diabetes or depression alone [36]. In a study of 12 643 Hungarian adults, individuals with comorbid depression and diabetes had significantly greater odds of prolonged bed days due to illness ($\geq$20 days) (OR 2.6, 95% CI 1.69–3.88), prolonged hospital stays ($\geq$18 days) (OR 2.1, 95% CI 1.27–3.45) and multiple hospital admissions (OR 2.8, 95% CI 1.13–2.82) compared to those with diabetes alone [37].

## MEDICAL COSTS OF COEXISTING DIABETES AND DEPRESSION

Multiple studies have established that the coexistence of diabetes and depression is associated with increased healthcare use and healthcare costs. Ciechanowski *et al.* [38] studied 367 subjects with diabetes and found that people with depression had almost a twofold increase in healthcare cost compared to people without depression (unadjusted

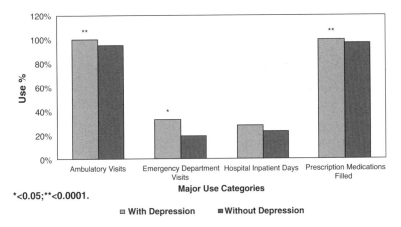

**Figure 3.1**   Pattern of healthcare use among diabetic persons with and without depression, United States 1996.

six-month total healthcare cost $3654 vs $2094). In another study of 825 subjects with diabetes, Egede *et al.* [39] assessed US population weighted healthcare cost and found a 4.5-fold higher cost in people with depression compared to those without depression ($247 million vs $55 million). For this chapter, data from that study were reanalysed to examine the percentage use across different use categories by depression status (Figure 3.1) as well as median cost across multiple cost categories by depression status (Figure 3.2). This reanalysis provides a better graphic display of the impact of depression on patterns of use and cost in adults with type 2 diabetes.

Finkelstein *et al.* [40] analysed Medicare claims data in elderly subjects with diabetes and found that those with depression had twofold increased healthcare cost compared to those without depression ($25 360 vs $10 358). Gilmer *et al.* [41] used claims data to calculate three-year healthcare cost in 1694 adults with diabetes. Standardized costs for those with depression were significantly higher than costs for those without depression ($31 967 vs 21 609).

In a study of 55 972 adults with diabetes, Le *et al.* [42] found that patients with diabetes and depression had higher diabetes-related medical costs ($3264) than patients with diabetes alone ($1297). They also found that depressed patients with diabetes had higher total medical costs ($19 298) than patients without depression ($4819). Kalsekar *et al.* [43] assessed health use and cost in 4294 adults with

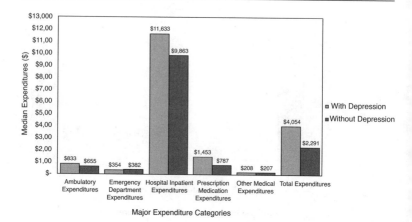

**Figure 3.2** Comparison of median expenditures between depressed and non-depressed persons with diabetes, United States 1996.

type 2 diabetes enrolled in Medicaid from 1998 to 2001 and found that patients with comorbid depression incurred a higher number of physician visits, emergency department visits, inpatient stays and prescription use and had 65% higher overall healthcare costs compared to those without depression. Nichols *et al.* [44] found that, in adjusted analyses, individuals with diabetes and minor depression used more ambulatory care visits and prescriptions than non-depressed adults, even though depression alone was not associated with higher resource use. Simon *et al.* [45] examined medical costs associated with depression in over 4000 patients with diabetes enrolled in a health maintenance organization: at every level of diabetes complications, major depression was associated with 50–100% greater medical costs. These studies confirm that comorbid depression is associated with increased healthcare costs in people with diabetes.

To provide updated national estimates of the medical cost of coexisting depression and diabetes in the United States, data from a nationally representative survey of the adult population from 2006 were analysed. The Medical Expenditure Panel Survey (MEPS) is cosponsored by the Agency for Healthcare Research and Quality (AHRQ) and the National Center for Health Statistics. It provides nationally representative estimates of healthcare use and expenditures for the civilian non-institutionalized US population. Data for the entire period of eligibility in 2006 were available for 32 577 individuals [46, 47]. The 2006 MEPS has two major components, the household component and the insurance component. The household component provides data from individual households and their members, which is supplemented by data from their medical providers. The insurance component collects detailed information for each person in the household on demographic characteristics, health conditions, health status, medical services use, charges and source of payments, access to care, satisfaction with care, health insurance coverage, income and employment [46, 47].

For this analysis, individuals were classified into four mutually exclusive diabetes and depression categories as follows: no diabetes and no depression, diabetes alone, depression alone, and diabetes and depression. The diagnosis of diabetes was based on self-report, while that of depression was based on a positive score for the two-item depression screen used in the 2006 MEPS [46, 47]. Population means for use and costs across multiple categories were compared for the four categories of depression and diabetes with the software for statistical analysis of correlated data, SUDAAN [48], to account for the complex survey design of MEPS. P-values were determined for the comparison of the diabetes only and the diabetes and depression groups to identify the incremental change in use and cost due to depression in adults with diabetes in the USA in 2006. The results show that individuals with diabetes and depression had greater use and cost for almost all categories examined (Table 3.1).

## COSTS OF TREATMENT OF COEXISTING DIABETES AND DEPRESSION

Studies of the economics of treatments of depressed individuals with diabetes have yielded positive results. A subgroup analysis of 418 patients with diabetes from the Improving Mood-Promoting Access to Collaborative (IMPACT) randomized controlled trial showed that depression intervention patients experienced 115 more depression-free days over 24 months, incremental cost per quality-adjusted life year ranged from $198 to $397, and incremental net benefit was $1129 dollars [49]. In another study of the cost effectiveness of treatment

**Table 3.1** Mean healthcare use and expenditures by diabetes and depression status, United States 2006

| | No Diabetes, No Depression N = 16 587 | Diabetes Only N = 1545 | Depression Only N = 1779 | Diabetes and Depression N = 395 |
|---|---|---|---|---|
| **Healthcare Use** | | | | |
| Total Dental Visits | 1.04 (1.00, 1.08) | 1.09 (0.98, 1.21) | 0.83 (0.73, 0.93) | 0.78[a] (0.59, 0.98) |
| Total ER Visits | 0.17 (0.16, 0.18) | 0.26 (0.23, 0.30) | 0.38 (0.33, 0.43) | 0.71[a] (0.55, 0.87) |
| Total Inpatient Stays | 0.09 (0.08, 0.10) | 0.23 (0.20, 0.26) | 0.21 (0.17, 0.24) | 0.41[a] (0.31, 0.52) |
| Total Office-Based Visits | 5.19 (4.99, 5.39) | 10.97 (10.05, 11.89) | 8.67 (7.87, 9.47) | 15.79[a] (13.54, 18.04) |
| Total Hospital Outpatient Visits | 0.43 (0.39, 0.47) | 1.38 (0.88, 1.87) | 1.10 (0.84, 1.35) | 2.09 (1.20, 2.98) |
| **Healthcare Expenditures** | | | | |
| Total ER Facility Expenditure | 100.94 (91.26, 110.62) | 190.35 (138.75, 241.95) | 209.99 (142.09, 277.90) | 374.25[a] (222.98, 525.51) |
| Total ER SBD Expenditure | 23.25 (20.59, 25.90) | 40.41 (30.79, 50.04) | 44.05 (30.41, 57.69) | 74.69[a] (51.25, 98.12) |
| Total Inpatient Facility Expenditure | 753.99 (659.63, 848.35) | 2387.50 (1865.24, 2909.76) | 1575.18 (1198.89, 1951.46) | 4208.29[a] (2898.61, 5517.97) |

| | | | |
|---|---|---|---|
| Total Inpatient SBD Expenditure | 135.65 (121.85, 149.44) | 327.81 (256.33, 399.29) | 259.93 (195.10, 324.75) | 555.14$^a$ (365.79, 744.49) |
| Total Office-Based Expenditure | 855.13 (806.22, 904.04) | 1998.64 (1772.42, 2224.85) | 1457.10 (1191.72, 1722.48) | 2675.11$^a$ (2060.79, 3289.43) |
| Total Hospital Outpatient Expenditure | 254.23 (224.54, 283.91) | 631.30 (494.35, 768.26) | 486.37 (344.43, 628.30) | 819.48 (530.66, 1108.30) |
| Total Home Health Agency Expenditure | 71.17 (52.49, 89.85) | 439.49 (188.49, 690.49) | 230.82 (155.18, 306.45) | 1135.06$^a$ (612.99, 1657.13) |
| Total Prescription Expenditure | 690.83 (627.12, 754.54) | 3006.03 (2767.49, 3244.57) | 1515.55 (1379.32, 1651.78) | 4008.99$^a$ (3540.05, 4477.93) |
| **Total Expenditure** | | | | |
| Total Healthcare Expenditure | 3297.80 (3138.66, 3456.93) | 9582.14 (8726.93, 10437.35) | 6263.41 (5629.98, 6896.85) | 14530.99$^a$ (12231.88, 16830.10) |

SBD – separately billing doctor. SBD expenses typically cover services provided to patients in hospital settings by providers like radiologists, anaesthesiologists and pathologists, whose charges are often not included in hospital bills.

ER – Emergency Room.

[a] Significant p-value ($p < 0.05$) for comparisons of diabetes and depression to diabetes only groups.

of depression among individuals with diabetes, Simon *et al.* [50] concluded that systematic depression treatment significantly increased time free of depression, resulting in an economic benefit from the perspective of the health plan. Patients who received the systematic depression treatment accumulated a mean of 61 additional days free of depression (95% CI 11–82 days) and had, on average, $314 less costs associated with outpatient services. The net economic benefit was $952 per treated patient when each day free of depression was valued at $10 [47].

In the Pathways depression intervention program, Katon *et al.* [51] compared the depression intervention group to usual care and found that patients in the intervention arm of the study experienced improved depression outcomes and reduced five-year mean costs of $3907 compared to patients in the usual source of the care arm.

In summary, these studies suggest that treatment of depression in people with diabetes is both efficacious and cost effective and can result in improved overall diabetes outcomes.

## AREAS FOR FUTURE RESEARCH

Based on the literature reviewed above, there is little doubt that coexisting depression increases resource use and cost in adults with diabetes. However, there are three main questions that have not been answered adequately.

Firstly, does the impact of depression on health use and cost differ for type 1 and type 2 diabetes? Most of the studies reviewed in this chapter did not differentiate between type 1 and type 2 diabetes, so it is difficult to estimate the economic burden of depression in type 1 diabetes. Future studies need to include sufficient samples of type 1 and type 2 patients and use the same methodology to allow direct comparisons.

Secondly, what are the independent predictors of increased healthcare use and cost in people with diabetes and comorbid depression? Multiple studies have shown that, among people with diabetes, depression is more prevalent in those with two or more coexisting chronic conditions [12] and is associated with treatment non-adherence [52], medication non-adherence [53], increased complications [54] and decreased quality of care [55]. However, few studies have attempted to identify how these factors contribute to increased health use and cost, and whether interventions directed at some of these factors can lead to decreases in patterns of use and/or cost. Garrison *et al.* [56] found that internalizing disorders were associated with about 1.8-fold increased odds of rehospitalization after an index admission for diabetes among adolescents aged 13–18 years. However, no significant association was found for children aged 5–12 years. Further studies are needed to clarify the independent predictors of increased health use and cost in individuals with type 1 and type 2 diabetes, preferably using a longitudinal design.

Thirdly, what is the full cost of illness for diabetes and comorbid depression? Currently, there are no studies that assess direct and indirect costs of illness for diabetes and coexisting depression. Direct cost of illness studies typically underestimate the true economic burden of an illness, so comprehensive studies are needed to assess the direct medical and indirect (e.g. disability, work loss and premature mortality) costs for diabetes and comorbid depression. There are sufficient data from multiple individual studies to come up with valid assumptions and reliable estimates of the total burden of depression in individuals with diabetes. These types of studies are urgently needed to assist policy makers in resource allocation, especially in the current era of fragmented care.

## REFERENCES

1. International Diabetes Federation (2009) Diabetes Atlas,  4th edn, www.diabetesatlas.org.
2. National Institute of Diabetes and Digestive and Kidney Diseases (2008) National Diabetes Statistics, 2007 Fact Sheet. US Department of Health and Human Services, National Institutes of Health, Bethesda.
3. Greden, J.F. (2003) Physical symptoms of depression: unmet needs. *J. Clin. Psychiatry*, **64** (Suppl. 7), 5–11.
4. World Health Organization (2005) Revised global burden of disease (GBD) 2002 estimates,  www.who.int.
5. Ustun, T.B., Ayuso-Mateos, J.L., Chatterji, S. *et al.* (2004) Global burden of depressive disorders in the year 2000. *Br. J. Psychiatry*, **184**, 386–392.

6. Kessler, R.C., Berglund, P., Demler, O. *et al.* (2003) The epidemiology of major depressive disorder: results from the National Comorbidity Survey Replication (NCS-R). *JAMA*, **289**, 3095–3105.

7. Alonso, J., Angermeyer, M.C., Bernert, S. *et al.* (2004) Prevalence of mental disorders in Europe: results from the European Study of the Epidemiology of Mental Disorders (ESEMeD) project. *Acta Psychiatr. Scand.*, **109** (Suppl. 420), 21–27.

8. Demyttenaere, K., Bruffaerts, R., Posada-Villa, J. *et al.* (2004) Prevalence, severity, and unmet need for treatment of mental disorders in the World Health Organization World Mental Health Surveys. *JAMA*, **291**, 2581–2590.

9. Michaud, C.M., Murray, C.J., and Bloom, B.R. (2001) Burden of disease – implications for future research. *JAMA*, **285**, 535–539.

10. US Department of Health and Human Services (1999) Mental health: a report of the Surgeon General. US Department of Health and Human Services, Rockville.

11. Egede, L.E. and Zheng, D. (2003) Independent factors associated with major depressive disorder in a national sample of individuals with diabetes. *Diabetes Care*, **26**, 104–111.

12. Egede, L.E. (2005) Effect of comorbid chronic diseases on prevalence and odds of depression in adults with diabetes. *Psychosom. Med.*, **67**, 46–51.

13. Anderson, R.J., Freedland, K.E., Clouse, R.E., and Lustman, P.J. (2001) The prevalence of comorbid depression in adults with diabetes: a meta-analysis. *Diabetes Care*, **24**, 1069–1078.

14. Lin, E.H., Korff, M.V., Alonso, J. *et al.* (2008) Mental disorders among persons with diabetes – results from the World Mental Health Surveys. *J. Psychosom. Res.*, **65**, 571–580.

15. Li, C., Ford, E.S., Strine, T.W. *et al.* (2008) Prevalence of depression among U.S. adults with diabetes: findings from the 2006 behavioral risk factor surveillance system. *Diabetes Care*, **31**, 105–107.

16. Li, C., Ford, E.S., Zhao, G. *et al.* (2009) Prevalence and correlates of undiagnosed depression among U.S. adults with diabetes: the Behavioral Risk Factor Surveillance System 2006. *Diabetes Res. Clin. Pract.*, **83**, 268–279.

17. Kogan, S.M., Brody, G.H., Crawley, C. *et al.* (2007) Correlates of elevated depressive symptoms among rural African American adults with type 2 diabetes. *Ethn. Dis.*, **17**, 106–112.

18. Gary, T.L., Crum, R.M., Cooper-Patrick, L. *et al.* (2000) Depressive symptoms and metabolic control in African-Americans with type 2 diabetes. *Diabetes Care*, **23**, 23–29.

19. Mier, N., Bocanegra-Alonso, A., Zhan, D. *et al.* (2008) Clinical depressive symptoms and diabetes in a binational border population. *J. Am. Board Fam. Med.*, **21**, 223–233.

20. Asghar, S., Hussain, A., Ali, S.M. *et al.* (2007) Prevalence of depression and diabetes: a population-based study from rural Bangladesh. *Diabet. Med.*, **24**, 872–877.

21. Sotiropoulos, A., Papazafiropoulou, A., Apostolou, O. *et al.* (2008) Prevalence of depressive symptoms among non insulin treated Greek type 2 diabetic subjects. *BMC Res. Notes*, **1**, 101.

22. Zahid, N., Asghar, S., Claussen, B., and Hussain, A. (2008) Depression and diabetes in a rural community in Pakistan. *Diabetes Res. Clin. Pract.*, **79**, 124–127.

23. Almawi, W., Tamim, H., Al-Sayed, N. *et al.* (2008) Association of comorbid depression, anxiety, and stress disorders with Type 2 diabetes in Bahrain, a country with a very high prevalence of Type 2 diabetes. *J. Endocrinol. Invest.*, **31**, 1020–1024.

24. Khamseh, M.E., Baradaran, H.R., and Rajabali, H. (2007) Depression and diabetes in Iranian patients: a comparative study. *Int. J. Psychiatry Med.*, **37**, 81–86.

25. Ali, S., Stone, M.A., Peters, J.L. *et al.* (2006) The prevalence of comorbid depression in adults with Type 2 diabetes: a systematic review and meta-analysis. *Diabet. Med.*, **23**, 1165–1173.

26. Greenberg, P.E., Stiglin, L.E., Finkelstein, S.N., and Berndt, E.R. (1993) The economic burden of depression in 1990. *J. Clin. Psychiatry*, **54**, 405–418.

27. Druss, B.G. and Rosenheck, R.A. (1999) Patterns of health care costs associated with depression and substance abuse in a national sample. *Psychiatr. Serv.*, **50**, 214–218.

28. Druss, B.G., Rosenheck, R.A., and Sledge, W.H. (2000) Health and disability costs of depressive illness in a major U.S. corporation. *Am. J. Psychiatry*, **157**, 1274–1278.

29. Druss, B.G., Marcus, S.C., Olfson, M. *et al.* (2001) Comparing the national economic burden of five chronic conditions. *Health Aff.*, **20**, 233–241.

30. Chan, A.L., Yang, T.C., Chen, J.X. *et al.* (2006) Cost of depression of adults in Taiwan. *Int. J. Psychiatry Med.*, **36**, 131–135.

31. Hu, T.W., He, Y., Zhang, M., and Chen, N. (2007) Economic costs of depression in China. *Soc. Psychiatry Psychiatr. Epidemiol.*, **42**, 110–116.

32. Unutzer, J., Schoenbaum, M., Katon, W.J. *et al.* (2009) Healthcare costs associated with depression in medically ill fee-for-service Medicare participants. *J. Am. Geriatr. Soc.*, **57**, 506–510.

33. Black, S.A., Markides, K.S., and Ray, L.A. (2003) Depression predicts increased incidence of adverse health outcomes in older Mexican Americans with type 2 diabetes. *Diabetes Care*, **26**, 2822–2828.
34. Egede, L.E. (2004) Diabetes, major depression, and functional disability among U.S. adults. *Diabetes Care*, **27**, 421–428.
35. Egede, L.E. (2004) Effects of depression on work loss and disability bed days in individuals with diabetes. *Diabetes Care*, **27**, 1751–1753.
36. Goldney, R.D., Phillips, P.J., Fisher, L.J., and Wilson, D.H. (2004) Diabetes, depression, and quality of life: a population study. *Diabetes Care*, **27**, 1066–1070.
37. Vamos, E.P., Mucsi, I., Keszei, A. *et al.* (2009) Comorbid depression is associated with increased healthcare utilization and lost productivity in persons with diabetes: a large nationally representative Hungarian population survey. *Psychosom. Med.*, **71**, 501–507.
38. Ciechanowski, P.S., Katon, W.J., and Russo, J.E. (2000) Depression and diabetes: impact of depressive symptoms on adherence, function, and costs. *Arch. Intern. Med.*, **160**, 3278–3285.
39. Egede, L.E., Zheng, D., and Simpson, K. (2002) Comorbid depression is associated with increased health care use and expenditures in individuals with diabetes. *Diabetes Care*, **25**, 464–470.
40. Finkelstein, E.A., Bray, J.W., Chen, H. *et al.* (2003) Prevalence and costs of major depression among elderly claimants with diabetes. *Diabetes Care*, **26**, 415–420.
41. Gilmer, T.P., O'Connor, P.J., Rush, W.A. *et al.* (2005) Predictors of health care costs in adults with diabetes. *Diabetes Care*, **28**, 59–64.
42. Le, T.K., Able, S.L., and Lage, M.J. (2006) Resource use among patients with diabetes, diabetic neuropathy, or diabetes with depression. *Cost Eff. Resour. Alloc.*, **4**, 18.
43. Kalsekar, I.D., Madhavan, S.M., Amonkar, M.M. *et al.* (2006) The effect of depression on health care utilization and costs in patients with type 2 diabetes. *Manag. Care Interface*, **19**, 39–46.
44. Nichols, L., Barton, P.L., Glazner, J., and McCollum, M. (2007) Diabetes, minor depression and health care utilization and expenditures: a retrospective database study. *Cost Eff. Resour. Alloc.*, **5**, 4.
45. Simon, G.E., Katon, W.J., Lin, E.H. *et al.* (2005) Diabetes complications and depression as predictors of health service costs. *Gen. Hosp. Psychiatry*, **27**, 344–351.
46. Agency for Healthcare Research and Quality (2008) The Medical Expenditure Panel Survey. 2006 Full Year Consolidated Data File (Documentation). Agency for Healthcare Research and Quality, Rockville.

47. Agency for Healthcare Research and Quality (2008) The Medical Expenditure Panel Survey. 2006 Full Year Consolidated Data File (Code Book). Agency for Healthcare Research and Quality, Rockville.
48. Research Triangle Institute (2001) Software for Statistical Analysis of Correlated Data (SUDAAN), Release 9.0.1. Research Triangle Institute, Research Triangle Park.
49. Katon, W., Unutzer, J., Fan, M.Y. *et al.* (2006) Cost-effectiveness and net benefit of enhanced treatment of depression for older adults with diabetes and depression. *Diabetes Care*, **29**, 265–270.
50. Simon, G.E., Katon, W.J., Lin, E.H. *et al.* (2007) Cost-effectiveness of systematic depression treatment among people with diabetes mellitus. *Arch. Gen. Psychiatry*, **64**, 65–72.
51. Katon, W.J., Russo, J.E., Von Korff, M. *et al.* (2008) Long-term effects on medical costs of improving depression outcomes in patients with depression and diabetes. *Diabetes Care*, **31**, 1155–1159.
52. Gonzalez, J.S., Peyrot, M., McCarl, L.A. *et al.* (2008) Depression and diabetes treatment nonadherence: a meta-analysis. *Diabetes Care*, **31**, 2398–2403.
53. DiMatteo, M.R., Lepper, H.S., and Croghan, T.W. (2000) Depression is a risk factor for noncompliance with medical treatment: meta-analysis of the effects of anxiety and depression on patient adherence. *Arch. Intern. Med.*, **160**, 2101–2107.
54. de Groot, M., Anderson, R., Freedland, K.E. *et al.* (2001) Association of depression and diabetes complications: a meta-analysis. *Psychosom. Med.*, **63**, 619–630.
55. Egede, L.E., Ellis, C., and Grubaugh, A.L. (2009) The effect of depression on self-care behaviors and quality of care in a national sample of adults with diabetes. *Gen. Hosp. Psychiatry*, **31**, 422–427.
56. Garrison, M.M., Katon, W.J., and Richardson, L.P. (2005) The impact of psychiatric comorbidities on readmissions for diabetes in youth. *Diabetes Care*, **28**, 2150–2154.

# CHAPTER 4

# Treatment of Depression in Patients with Diabetes: Efficacy, Effectiveness and Maintenance Trials, and New Service Models

**Wayne Katon**

*Department of Psychiatry and Behavioral Sciences, University of Washington School of Medicine, Seattle, WA, USA*

**Christina van der Feltz-Cornelis**

*Department of Clinical and Developmental Psychology, University of Tilburg; Centre of Top Clinical Care for Somatoform Disorder, GGZ Breburg, Breda; Trimbos Institute, Utrecht, The Netherlands*

Two systematic reviews have found rates of major depression to be between 12 and 17% in patients with diabetes [1, 2]. These rates have been shown to be twofold higher than those of medical controls [1, 2]. Patients with comorbid major depression and diabetes, compared to those with diabetes alone, have been shown to have a higher medical symptom burden [3], more decrements in functioning and quality of life [4], higher medical costs [5], poor self-care (i.e. adherence to diet, exercise, cessation of smoking recommendations and disease control medication) [6], poorer glycaemic control [7], an increased number

*Depression and Diabetes* Edited by Wayne Katon, Mario Maj and Norman Sartorius
© 2010 John Wiley & Sons, Ltd

of Framingham risk factors for cardiovascular disease [8], and an increased risk of macrovascular and microvascular complications and mortality [9–11].

Depression tends to be either a chronic or a recurrent condition in patients with diabetes. Data from a large study of over 4800 patients with diabetes enrolled in a health maintenance organization (HMO) found that approximately 70% of those with comorbid depression (based on scoring ≥10 on the Patient Health Questionnaire-9) had experienced affective symptoms for two years or longer [12]. Among mixed-aged depressed patients without diabetes in this same health maintenance organization, only approximately 20% described two or more years of affective symptoms [13]. The increase in chronicity of depression is, at least in part, age related. Patients with diabetes tend to be older, and recent primary care data have shown that the average length of an episode of depression in older primary care patients is approximately 18 months [14], whereas in mixed-aged populations the mean length of an episode is approximately 4–6 months [15].

The tendency for depressive symptoms to be chronic in patients with diabetes is also shown by recent data from a five-year follow-up study of approximately 2700 patients with diabetes. Approximately 82% of patients who met DSM-IV criteria for major depression at five-year follow-up had minor or major depression at baseline [16]. Finally, the recurrent course of depression was shown in a longitudinal study, which found that 79% of patients with diabetes who had major depression relapsed over a five-year follow-up period, with a mean of four episodes per patient [17].

A recent large European study showed that over 50% of community respondents with anxiety and depressive disorders were not receiving healthcare services for their psychiatric illness, whereas only 8% of respondents with diabetes reported no use of services for their medical condition [18]. Thus, the current unmet need for mental health care is significantly higher than the unmet need for medical care. Given that the vast majority of patients with diabetes are receiving regular medical care, it is possible that patients with comorbid depression and diabetes would receive more accurate diagnosis and effective treatment for depression than those with depression alone. However, in a large United States population-based sample, over a 12-month period, only approximately 51% of patients with major depression and diabetes were accurately recognized by the healthcare system [19]. Factors associated with higher recognition rates included female gender, comorbid dysthymia or panic attacks, the patient's perception of poor health, and making more than seven primary care visits per year [19]. Among those whose depression was accurately diagnosed, there were deficits in quality of care, with 43% receiving one or more antidepressant prescriptions and only 6.7% receiving four or more sessions of psychotherapy during the 12-month period [19]. The likelihood is that patients with fee-for-service medical insurance in the United States would have even lower rates of detection and provision of guideline-level depression care, due to more financial, geographic and organizational barriers to mental health care.

Given the high prevalence and chronicity of depression in patients with diabetes and the adverse impact of depression on functioning, quality of life and medical outcomes, the provision of evidence-based depression treatment is of great public health importance. This chapter focuses on: (a) whether research-proven pharmacotherapies and psychotherapies are efficacious in patients with comorbid depression and diabetes; (b) the development and testing of primary care-based health services models to improve detection and quality of depression care for this population; and (c) the evidence about maintenance depression treatment.

Steps are also described to enhance diagnosis and engagement of patients with diabetes in depression treatment as well as the necessary changes in primary care systems needed to enhance early accurate diagnosis and provision of evidence-based treatments for affective illness. Finally, new research models that combine care management for depression with care management to improve glycaemic, lipid and blood pressure control in patients with diabetes and/or heart disease are described.

## EFFICACY STUDIES

Most large treatment studies have found that medical illness and decrements in physical functioning are associated with lower rates of response to evidence-based depression treatments [20]. Patients with diabetes frequently develop complications of their illness that lead to decrements in functioning, such as neuropathy, peripheral ulcers and amputation. Recent US Medicare data have shown that approximately 70% of patients with diabetes have four or more comorbid medical conditions and these patients with multiple conditions often have the most deficits in functioning and high rates of comorbid depression [21]. Therefore, an important question for researchers and clinicians is whether evidence-based pharmacotherapies and psychotherapies that have proven effective in populations of patients with depression with minimal medical illness would be as efficacious in patients with diabetes.

Several systematic reviews have been completed exploring effect sizes of psychotherapeutic as well as pharmacological treatments of patients with comorbid depression and diabetes [22, 23]. Efficacy trials generally evaluate intensive treatment of a carefully selected patient group by highly trained staff. Patients with clinically significant psychiatric comorbidities, such as panic disorder or medical comorbidities, are often excluded from these trials.

A systematic review of efficacy trials performed in 2009 yielded 11 randomized clinical trials, five on psychotherapeutic interventions and six on pharmacological treatments [24–34]. The results of this review are shown in Table 4.1. Most trials were small, with only one recruiting more than 100 patients and the others including 60 or fewer patients. Most trials were completed on patients with type 2 diabetes with serious depressive symptoms or major depressive disorder, and effect sizes were specified for depressive symptom severity as well as for glycaemic control.

The results were presented in terms of standardized effect sizes (Cohen's $d$). These effect sizes indicate by how many standard units the intervention group is better off than the control group on a depression severity scale. The effect size ($d$) is usually calculated by subtracting the average score of the control group from the average score of the experimental group and dividing the raw difference score by the pooled standard deviation of the experimental and control group [35]. An effect size of 0.5 thus indicates that the mean of the experimental group is half a standard unit larger than the mean of the control group. It is generally assumed that an effect size of 0.56–1.2 represents a large clinical effect,

**Table 4.1** Efficacy trials of psychotherapeutic and pharmacological treatments for depression in patients with diabetes

| Study | N (completers); diabetes type; mean age | Intervention conditions; follow-up (FU) | Outcome assessment (depression; diabetes, DM) | Effect size (depression; diabetes, DM) | Comments |
|---|---|---|---|---|---|
| *Psychotherapeutic interventions (N = 310)* | | | | | |
| Lustman et al., 1998 (USA) [24] | N = 41; 1C0% type 2; 53.1–56.4 ± 10.5–9.7 | CBT plus diabetes education versus diabetes education alone FU: 11 wk, 6 mo | *Depression:* Response (reduction BDI ≥ 50%) $p < 0.001$ in CBT group *DM:* HbA1c lower in CBT group, $p < 0.03$ | *Depression:* $\Delta$ −1.112 *DM:* $\Delta$ −0.704 | Improvement in depression as well as glycaemic control in CBT group |
| Huang et al., 2002 (China) [25] | N = 59; 100% type 2; N/A | Antidiabetics + diabetic education + psychological treatment + relaxation and music treatment vs antidiabetics only FU: 3 mo | *Depression:* SDS total score difference in means 0.07, $p < 0.05$ *DM:* HbA1c difference in means 1.7, $p < 0.05$ | *Depression:* $\Delta$ −0.521 *DM:* $\Delta$ −0.521 | Improvement in depression as well as glycaemic control in group treated with psychotherapy |

*(Continued)*

**Table 4.1** (Continued)

| Study | N (completers); diabetes type; mean age | Intervention conditions; follow-up (FU) | Outcome assessment (depression; diabetes, DM) | Effect size (depression; diabetes, DM) | Comments |
|---|---|---|---|---|---|
| Li et al., 2003 (China) [26] | N = 120; N/A; 50.5–52.3 ± 10.4–11.2 | Antidiabetics + diabetic education + psychological treatment vs antidiabetics only FU: 4 wk | *Depression:* SDS total score difference in means 13.4, p < 0.01 *DM:* FBG difference in means 2.09, p < 0.05 | *Depression:* Δ −0.478 *DM:* Δ −0.362 | Anxiety (SAS ≥ 50) taken into account as well. Improvement in depression as well as glycaemic control in group treated with psychotherapy |
| Lu et al., 2005 (China) [27] | N = 60; 100% type 2; 65.6–64.9 ± 9.8–9.5 | Diabetes and CVA education + electromyographic treatment + psychological treatment vs usual care FU: 4 wk | *Depression:* HAMD-17 total score difference in means 7.3, p < 0.01 *DM:* difference in means FPG 1.54, p < 0.05 | *Depression:* Δ −0.688 *DM:* Δ −0.517 | Hemiplegia after CVA as DM complication. Improvement in depression as well as glycaemic control in group treated with psychotherapy |

| Study | Sample | Intervention | Outcome | Effect size | Comments |
|---|---|---|---|---|---|
| Simson et al., 2008 (Germany) [28] | N = 30; 8C% Type 2; 6C.5 ± 10.9 | Individual supportive psychotherapy vs usual care FU: discharge (3–20 wk) | *Depression* HADS depression scale total score mean difference 1.9, p = 0.018 *DM*: PAID mean difference 7.6, p = 0.008 | *Depression:* Δ −0.918 *DM*: Δ −1.043 | Diabetic foot as DM complication. Improvement in depression as well as glycaemic control in supportive psychotherapy group |
| *Pharmacological interventions (N = 215)* | | | | | |
| Lustman et al., 1997 (USA) [29] | N = 28; 50% type 2; 49.0–49.2 ± 12.1–13.7 | Glucometertraining + nortriptyline vs placebo FU: 9 wk | *Depression:* BDI total score, mean difference 5.6, p = 0.03 *DM*: HbA1c, no significant difference, no outcome reported | Depression: Δ −0.868 *DM*: Δ 0 | Poorly controlled (HbA1c ≥9%) as inclusion criterion. Improvement in depression but not in glycaemic control in nortriptyline vs control. Nortrypitiline may have negative impact on glycemic control. *(Continued)* |

**Table 4.1** (Continued)

| Study | N (completers); diabetes type; mean age | Intervention conditions; follow-up (FU) | Outcome assessment (depression; diabetes, DM) | Effect size (depression; diabetes, DM) | Comments |
|---|---|---|---|---|---|
| Lustman et al., 2000 (USA) [30] | N = 54; 55.6% type 2; 45.0–47.7 ± 13.0–11.5 | Fluoxetine vs placebo FU: 8 wk | *Depression:* HAMD total score mean difference 26.7, p < 0.04 *DM:* HbA1c mean difference 0.33, p = 0.13 (n.s.) | *Depression:* Δ −0.573 *DM:* Δ 0.419 | Improvement in depression but not in glycaemic control in fluoxetine vs placebo. |
| Paile-Hyvärinen et al., 2003 (Finland) [31] | N = 13; 100% type 2; 61.1–62.3 ± 8.6–11.5 | Paroxetine vs placebo FU: 4 wk | After initial improvement in paroxetine group at 3 mo, no significant improvement for both outcomes at end of follow-up. *Depression:* MADRS total score mean difference 2.50, p = 0.25 | *Depression:* Δ −0.676 *DM:* Δ 1.073 | Poorly controlled (HbA1c ≥6.5% or FBG ≥7.0) as inclusion criterion. Probably a combination of ceiling effect and underpowered study. |

| Study | Sample | Intervention | Results | Effect size | Conclusion |
|---|---|---|---|---|---|
| Xue et al., 2004 (China) [32] | N = 48; 85.4% type 2 ; 21–65 | Paroxetine vs placebo FU: 8 wk | Depression: HAMD-17 total score mean difference 5.7, p < 0.01 DM: HbA1c mean difference 0.4, p = 0.245 (n.s.) DM: GHbA1c mean difference 0.37, p = 0.08 (n.s.) | Depression: Δ −0.776 DM: Δ 0.340 | Improvement in depression but not in glycaemic control in paroxetine vs placebo. |
| Gülseren et al., 2005 (Turkey) [33] | N = 23; 100% type 2; 58.2–57.1 ± 12.3–10.4 | Fluoxetine vs paroxetine FU: 12 wk | Both groups improved significantly in depression (HDRS mean difference 0.62, p = 0.003) but not in HbA1c (mean difference 0.11, n.s.) | | No significant difference between the two conditions. |

(Continued)

**Table 4.1** (*Continued*)

| Study | N (completers); diabetes type; mean age | Intervention conditions; follow-up (FU) | Outcome assessment (depression; diabetes, DM) | Effect size (depression; diabetes, DM) | Comments |
|---|---|---|---|---|---|
| Paile-Hyvärinen et al., 2007 (Finland) [34] | N = 49; 100% type 2; 59.5–59.2 ± 6.0–5.4 | Paroxetine vs placebo FU: 3 mo, 6 mo | *Depression:* HADS depression scale total score mean difference 0.7, p = 0.448 (n.s.) *DM:* GHbA1c mean difference 0.13, p = 0.693 (n.s.) | *Depression:* Δ −0.260 *DM:* Δ 0.135 | No significant improvement in depressive outcomes and glycaemic control. |

DM – diabetes; CBT – cognitive behavioural therapy; SDS – Self Rating Depression Scale; SAS – Zung Self Rating Anxiety Scale; HAMD-17 – Hamilton Depression Rating Scale – 17; FPG – fasting plasma glucose; CVA – cerebrovascular accident; HADS – Hospital Anxiety and Depression Scale; PAID – Problem Areas in Diabetes Survey; BDI – Beck Depression Inventory; MADRS – Montgomery–Asberg Depression Rating Scale; n.s. – not significant; N/A – not available.

while effect sizes of 0.33–0.55 are moderate and effect sizes of 0–0.32 are small [36].

As can be seen in Table 4.1, the effect sizes of the psychotherapeutic interventions were moderate to large for improvement of depressive symptoms, and moderate to large for improvement of glycaemic control. In a meta-analysis, the effect sizes of the psychotherapeutic trials were pooled. The pooled estimate of the psychotherapeutic trails was −0.645 (95% CI −0.874; −0.415) for depression outcomes, and −0.477 (95% −0.715; −0.239) for glycaemic control. Three of the five psychotherapy trials compared an evidence-based depression psychotherapy and diabetes education to diabetes education alone. Therefore, it is unclear whether improvements in glycaemic control were due to the beneficial effect of the depression-focused psychotherapy or the combination of both depression therapy and diabetes education.

As shown in Table 4.1, the pharmacotherapeutic interventions (all but one evaluated the efficacy of selective serotonin reuptake inhibitors, SSRIs) had moderate effects on depressive symptoms, and small effects on glycaemic control. The pooled estimate of the pharmacotherapeutic trials, of which only one (the Lustman study) included a direct intervention to improve glycaemic control, was −0.615 (95% CI −0.916, −0.313) for depression outcomes and −0.376 (95% −0.701; −0.052) for glycaemic control. The effect on depressive outcomes was very similar, but the effect on glycaemic control was smaller than that of the psychotherapeutic studies, many of which had explicit interventions aimed at improving glycaemic control. The pharmacologic trials were also small, with 13 to 54 patients enrolled. The small numbers of patients enrolled in both psychotherapy and pharmacologic efficacy trials limits the generalizability of the findings.

In terms of public health, the findings from the psychotherapy and pharmacotherapy trials suggest that, in order to improve self-care and glucose control in patients with diabetes and depression, simple treatment of the comorbid depressive disorder is likely to be insufficient. To improve both psychiatric and medical outcomes, a more comprehensive approach that includes both evidence-based depression treatment and interventions aimed at improving diabetes self-care and glucose control is likely to be needed.

## EFFECTIVENESS TRIALS: COLLABORATIVE DEPRESSION CARE

A key concept involved in the development of primary care-based models to improve care of chronic illnesses is population-based care [37]. This is an approach to planning and delivering care to defined patient populations which tries to ensure that effective interventions reach all patients that need them (i.e. all patients with diabetes who have comorbid major depression and/or dysthymia) [37]. This model often requires depression screening and a team approach to care rather than infrequent brief visits with a primary care physician. The model was developed to overcome the gaps in depression treatment experienced by patients with diabetes, with only 50% being accurately diagnosed and only half of these receiving even a minimal standard of pharmacologic or psychotherapeutic treatments [37].

Collaborative care is a population-based health services model that was developed to increase exposure of patients with depression in primary care systems to evidence-based depression pharmacologic care and psychotherapies [37]. The key components of collaborative care include: enhanced patient education using videotapes, pamphlets and books; integration of allied health professionals into primary care systems to track depression outcomes, side effects and adherence and to provide support for behavioural change; use of a monitoring tool such as the Patient Health Questionnaire – 9 (PHQ-9) [38] and an electronic disease register; caseload supervision by a psychiatrist; and stepped care approaches. Stepped care involves increasing the intensity of care based on persistent depressive symptoms.

In a study in The Netherlands, psychiatric consultation was found to facilitate implementation of stepped care for depressed patients [39]. A similar positive effect of psychiatric caseload supervision of the allied health professional who provided collaborative care was established in a meta-analytic review of 37 trials [40]. Thus, in a stepped care approach, if a patient initiates treatment with an evidence-based psychotherapy and remains depressed at 4–6 weeks, an antidepressant may be recommended during psychiatric supervision. Alternatively, if an initial trial of an antidepressant has not led to adequate symptom relief, the medication may be changed or augmented or psychotherapy added. Given the low rates of detection of depression among patients with diabetes, developing population-based models like collaborative care usually requires methods to screen patients for depression.

There are now three trials of collaborative care versus usual care in patients with depression and diabetes [12, 41, 42]. These studies were developed in distinct populations: mixed-aged patients enrolled in nine primary care clinics of a non-profit HMO [12]; elderly patients ($\geq$65 years of age) in eight systems of care in seven geographic regions of the United States [41]; and mixed-age, mainly Hispanic patients, mostly living below United States poverty levels and attending two large primary care clinics in Los Angeles [42]. In all three trials, the population of patients with diabetes in the primary care systems were screened for depression with a questionnaire and those with major depression and/or dysthymia were then offered randomization to either collaborative care or usual care [12, 41, 42]. These trials included representative patients from the population, only excluding those with terminal medical illness, dementia, or already seeing a psychiatrist. In two of the trials, approximately 50% of the randomized patients were taking an antidepressant but still met criteria for major depression or dysthymia and thus met inclusion criteria for the trial [12, 41].

All three collaborative care interventions offered a choice of starting with antidepressant medication or problem solving therapy (PST) [12, 41, 42]. Care managers worked in a team with the psychiatrist and primary care physician to provide enhanced education about depression, track symptoms, adherence and side effects, provide recommendations about medications to the primary care physicians based on caseload supervision by the psychiatrist, and provide PST. All three trials included a stepped care approach. Thus, if patients chose antidepressant medication as their initial treatment, but did not respond to optimal dosages, their antidepressant would be augmented or changed, or PST could be added. Similarly, if they did not respond to an initial treatment choice of PST, antidepressant medication could be added. These trials were focused on improving quality of care of depression and did not specifically focus on quality of care of diabetes.

All three trials showed significant improvements in quality of depression care compared to the usual care control groups, with improvement in percentage of patients treated with and adhering to antidepressant medication and the percentage receiving $\geq 4$ sessions of psychotherapy. All three trials also showed improvements in depressive symptoms compared to usual care over the initial 12- to 18-month period [12, 41, 42]. Two of the three trials included a 24-month follow-up and showed continued improvement in depressive symptoms compared to usual care at the 24-month stage (one year after the intervention ended) [12, 41]. Cohen's $d$ in terms of improvement of severity of depressive symptoms in the three trials was 0.320, 0.676 and 0.337, which can be considered moderate to large effects. In a meta-analysis, the pooled estimate of Cohen's $d$ for the three collaborative care trials was 0.441 (95% CI $-0.644$; $-0.251$).

Two of the three trials also showed improvement compared to usual care in physical functioning and quality of life over the initial 12- to 18-month period [12, 41, 42]. Thus, enhancing the quality of depression care appears to be an effective way to decrease physical decline in these aging medically ill populations. However, none of the three trials showed improvement in the collaborative care intervention group compared to the usual care controls in most components of self-care (i.e. adherence to checking blood glucose, diet, cessation of smoking, or taking disease control medication as prescribed) or mean $HbA_{1c}$ levels [12, 41–43]. These data are supported by several large trials of enhancing treatment of depression in patients with post-myocardial infarction, which have shown improvements in quality of depression care and depression outcomes, but not in cardiac complications or mortality [44, 45].

Two of the three collaborative care trials have completed cost-effectiveness analyses. These trials have shown that collaborative care versus usual primary care was associated with significant increments in depression-free days over a two-year period, that is, a total of 61 (95% CI 11, 82) and 115 (95% CI 72, 159) depression-free days, respectively [46, 47]. Both trials also showed that the (US)$500–700 increased mental health costs associated with the collaborative care intervention were offset by greater savings in total medical costs (Figure 4.1) [46, 47]. The medical cost savings were largely in year 2, emphasizing the importance of examining at least two years of healthcare cost data in these trials. Both trials showed a high probability that collaborative care was a 'dominant' intervention, defined as a medical intervention that is more effective and is

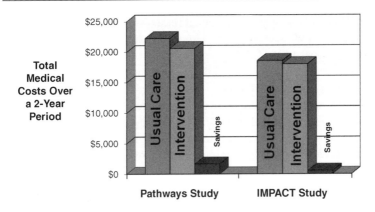

**Figure 4.1**  Healthcare costs of usual and collaborative (enhanced) care over a two-year period.

associated with medical cost savings [46, 47]. One of these trials also continued to track medical costs over a five-year period and found that the same trends for cost savings continued in years 3–5 in the intervention group compared to controls [48]. This suggests that enhancing depression care and outcomes in patients with depression and diabetes may place patients on a different long-term medical cost trajectory.

## MAINTENANCE TRIALS

Given the high rates of relapse and chronicity in patients with depression and diabetes that are described above, researchers have begun to test the effect of maintenance antidepressant treatment.

A recent maintenance trial randomized 152 patients who had recovered with an open label trial of sertraline to either sertraline or placebo for up to 52 weeks [49]. Patients who received maintenance treatment with the SSRI had a significantly greater depression-free interval compared to those treated with placebo (median time to recurrence was 57 days in the placebo group compared to 226 days in the patients treated with sertraline) [49]. There were no significant differences in glycaemic control between sertraline and placebo in this maintenance phase of treatment. However, both depression recovery with the SSRI as well as sustained remission with or without active treatments were associated with improvements in HbA$_{1c}$ levels for at least one year [49].

A second maintenance trial that treated 93 patients with type 2 diabetes with acute phase bupropion offered maintenance treatment with this medication to patients who remitted ($N = 63$) at the dosage that was associated with remission [50]. Body mass index (BMI), total fat mass and HbA$_{1c}$ values decreased significantly and composite diabetes care improved over the initial acute phase, and these effects persisted through the maintenance phase. Reduction in both BMI and depression severity with bupropion treatment predicted lower HbA$_{1c}$ levels after acute phase therapy, but only a reduction in depression predicted lower HbA$_{1c}$ levels during the maintenance phase of treatment [50].

The first two trials of collaborative care included a session of relapse prevention for patients who were nearing completion of the one-year intervention [12, 41]. The relapse prevention session included a review with the patient about prodromal symptoms (i.e. symptoms that are harbingers that they may be having relapse of depression) and strategies to cope with relapse, such as calling their primary care physician. The relapse prevention sessions also included stress reduction techniques the patient would regularly engage in, such as exercise and recommendations about maintenance antidepressant treatment or referral for more intensive psychotherapy. Both of these collaborative care trials showed that intervention patients were continuing to experience significantly less depressive symptoms compared to usual care controls one year after completing the 12-month trial [12, 41].

## NEW TREATMENT MODELS

Piette *et al.* [51] have proposed a model to explain how depression treatment may improve the outcomes of comorbid chronic disease, which they applied to diabetes. An adaptation of this model to indicate reciprocal adverse effects of comorbid chronic disease and depressive illness is described in Figure 4.2. In this model, effective treatment of depression may be more difficult because of the adverse health

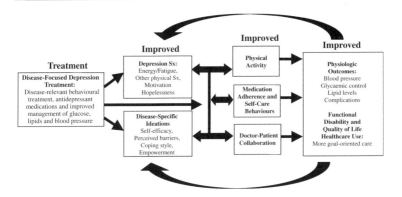

**Figure 4.2**    Adaptation of Piette's model linking depression and chronic disease outcomes. Reproduced with permission from Intellisphere, LLC

behaviours (smoking, obesity, sedentary lifestyle, lack of adherence to disease control medications) as well as higher symptom burden and functional disability associated with depression. Adverse health behaviours do not necessarily improve with effective depression treatment alone, and may be negative prognostic factors for depression outcomes (e.g. obesity is associated with negative social feedback, lower self-esteem and less exercise, which all effect mood). Sedentary lifestyle has been shown in prospective studies to be associated with subsequent development of depression [52]. Depression may also lead to poor self-care, resulting in a higher risk of diabetic macrovascular and microvascular complications, which in turn cause functional decrements which can precipitate a new episode or relapse of depression.

New treatment models (termed 'disease-focused depression treatment' in Figure 4.2) that focus on improving quality of both depression and medical treatment may be needed, which will emphasize improving depression treatment, increasing positive health behaviours (exercise and diet) and improving disease control of chronic medical illness by optimizing medication adherence and treatment in order to avoid complications. Several ongoing studies are testing these combined psychiatric and medical interventions in patients with diabetes and depression and those with diabetes and/or coronary heart disease and depression [53].

## IMPROVING DEPRESSION CARE IN INDIVIDUAL PATIENTS WITH DIABETES

Table 4.2 describes a clinical approach to assessing and treating depression and other psychiatric disorders in patients with diabetes [54]. Because of the high prevalence and adverse impact depression has in patients with diabetes, it is recommended that patients be screened for depression at least once a year with a tool such as the PHQ-9. The physician should have a high index of suspicion of a depression diagnosis in patients with poor control of blood glucose, poor adherence to self-care, pain and other somatic complaints and those who elicit frustration in the doctor–patient relationship. The PHQ-9 not only provides a probable diagnosis of major depression for those scoring $\geq 10$, but also includes a 0–27 severity score. This is an ideal scale for gauging success of treatment, and inclusion of the nine key symptoms of depression allows the practitioner to target treatment to specific symptoms, such as insomnia.

In a review, Gilbody *et al.* [55] found that screening for depression is effective if aimed at finding patients with sufficient severity of depressive symptoms to warrant treatment, and if appropriate treatment is subsequently offered as result of such a screening outcome. A similar outcome was found for combined screening for anxiety and depression [56]. Therefore, it is important to embed depression screening in a comprehensive treatment approach such as collaborative care.

Patients with depression and diabetes are frequently frustrated and demoralized and often present with physical symptoms. Depression is actually a better predictor of diabetes symptom reporting than is the level of $HbA_{1c}$ or the number of diabetes complications [3]. Patients are often uncertain about whether their diabetes and physical symptoms are causing depression or vice versa. They often feel resignation and guilt about not being able to manage their diabetic condition. Validating their sense of loss of control of their diabetes in a non-judgmental manner often allows the clinician to improve rapport and engagement [54]. It also offers the clinician the chance to provide education that the patient is experiencing two clinical diseases that can adversely impact each other and that both can be effectively treated. It is helpful to describe the maladaptive physical effects depression can have on medical symptom burden and diabetes control and to explore

**Table 4.2**    Improving depression care in patients with diabetes

*STEP 1 - Screen for:*

Depression with PHQ-9
Helplessness/'giving up' or sense of being overwhelmed about disease self-management
Comorbid panic attacks and PTSD with GAD-7
Inability to differentiate anxiety symptoms from diabetes symptoms (e.g. hypoglycaemia)
Associated eating concerns
Emotional eating in response to sadness/loneliness/anger
Binge eating/purging
Night eating

*STEP 2 - Improve self-management*

Explore 'loss of control' of disease self-management
Explore understanding of bidirectional link between stress and suboptimal disease self-management and outcomes
Define depression and how it overlaps with and is distinct from 'stress'
Review symptoms of depression and how these symptoms overlap with or mimic diabetes symptoms
Discuss depression-related medical symptom amplification
Break down tasks in self-management of diabetes, depression, heart disease, other illnesses
Help patient prioritize order of importance of specific tasks

*STEP 3 - Support*

Consider adjunctive brief psychotherapy for:
emotional eating (CBT)
breaking down problems (problem solving therapy)
improving treatment adherence (motivational interviewing)

*STEP 4 - Consider medication*

Comorbid depression and anxiety: SSRI or SNRI
Sexual dysfunction: use bupropion or if already responding to SSRI add buspirone 15 mg BID or bupropion SR 100 mg BID
Significant neuropathy: choose bupropion, venlafaxine or duloxetine due to effectiveness in treating neuropathic pain

PHQ-9 – Patient Health Questionnaire; PTSD – post-traumatic stress disorder; GAD-7 – Generalized Anxiety Disorder Assessment-7; CBT – cognitive behavioural therapy; SSRI – selective serotonin reuptake inhibitor; SNRI – serotonin-noradrenaline reuptake inhibitor.

how depression is affecting adherence to diet, exercise, checking blood glucose and taking medications as prescribed.

Many patients with depression also have comorbid anxiety disorders such as panic, generalized anxiety and post-traumatic stress disorder (PTSD). These disorders can also occur without comorbid depression and have been shown to maladaptively affect adherence and disease control in patients with diabetes [57, 58]. Therefore, screening for these disorders is also important. The Generalized Anxiety Disorder Assessment – 7 (GAD-7) is a new screening tool that screens for four potential anxiety disorders, that is, panic, PTSD, generalized anxiety disorder and social phobia [59].

Many patients with depressive and anxiety disorders and diabetes also go off diabetic diets and may binge on unhealthy foods when they feel emotionally vulnerable. Patients with diabetes also have higher rates of eating disorders. Carefully reviewing the changes in their dietary patterns associated with these stressful times in their life may help the clinician enhance understanding about the fluctuations in weight and glycaemic control that he/she is observing. Night eating syndrome, where the patient awakens during the night and often binges or snacks on unhealthy foods, has been shown to be associated with poor glucose control and diabetes complications [60]. Using motivational interviewing may help patients identify goals to begin to change dietary habits. Psychotherapy approaches, such as cognitive behavioural therapy, may be helpful for those with eating disorders.

A history of the common psychiatric and medical comorbidities or complications in patients with diabetes may lead to targeted selection of psychiatric medication. For patients with comorbid anxiety disorders, SSRIs and serotonin-noradrenaline reuptake inhibitors (SNRIs) may both help depression and effectively treat anxiety. Many patients with diabetes have sexual dysfunction due to the adverse effects of diabetes on the autonomic nervous and vascular systems. In these patients, bupropion is a reasonable first choice for treating depression because, unlike SSRIs or SNRIs, it does not adversely affect sexual function. For patients with depression and diabetic neuropathy, bupropion, venlafaxine and duloxetine may effectively treat both painful neuropathy and depression.

## CHANGES IN PRIMARY CARE SYSTEMS NECESSARY TO IMPROVE OUTCOMES OF PATIENTS WITH DEPRESSION AND DIABETES

The American Diabetes Association has now recommended screening for depression in patients with diabetes [61]. This recommendation has developed because of the research documenting the high prevalence of comorbid depression in diabetes and its adverse impact on symptom burden, self-care, functioning and diabetes complications. As reviewed above, valid and reliable screening tools like the PHQ-9 have been developed, but to begin screening requires linking this activity to changes in the primary care system to ensure both patient safety and improved quality of treatment and outcomes. For example, rapid evaluation of patients who score in the severe range on the PHQ-9 (a score of $\geq 20$) or those having suicidal ideation on the PHQ-9 is essential. This is similar to running medical tests and ensuring that the primary care system is set up to rapidly respond to a dangerously high laboratory value.

In one clinic that has set up PHQ-9 screening at the University of Washington, a nurse reviews all scores and any patient with a PHQ-9 score $\geq 20$ or rating the question about suicide ideation as more than half the days in the prior week receives an immediate social work referral. In collaborative care studies in The Netherlands, the PHQ-9 is monitored every two weeks, and in case of a positive score on the suicide question, the family physician is notified and the consultant psychiatrist consulted according to a protocol embedded in the electronic monitoring system [62, 63].

The collaborative care models that have been shown to improve quality and outcomes of depression patients with diabetes require a team approach. A depression care manager (DCM) and a psychiatrist are the two new members of the team. The DCM provides enhanced patient education about depression and careful tracking of PHQ-9 values, monitors side effects and adherence, and, based on psychiatric caseload supervision, provides recommendations about antidepressant medications to the primary care physician. When the patient continues to have persistent symptoms, the DCM facilitates referral back to the primary care physician or a potential consultation with the psychiatrist or referral for more intensive mental health screening. In some collaborative care studies, DCMs have also been trained to carry out brief psychotherapy, such as PST, in primary care. Psychiatric supervision of the depression case manager caseload is one of the most cost-effective components of the collaborative care model, because the psychiatrist can often supervise 100–200 cases per year. In some collaborative care models, the psychiatrist may also spend several hours a week evaluating patients with persistent depressive symptoms not improving with DCM and primary care treatment alone.

A key component of this model is either the development of a depression electronic registry to monitor visit dates, PHQ scores and type of treatment provided, or the integration of tracking of PHQ-9 scores into an existing diabetes registry. Many electronic registries have been developed using Access or Excel databases. In a new trial the Seattle research group has developed, termed the TEAMcare trial, PHQ-9 results have been integrated into a diabetes registry that monitors visit dates, LDL, blood pressure and $HbA_{1c}$ results [64].

These newer models of care, like TEAMcare, are using and training diabetes nurses to include depression screening and treatment as an important skill in overall diabetes care. In TEAMcare the diabetes nurses phase in treatment by first enhancing quality of depression care, then focusing on improving quality of care for blood pressure, lipids and glycaemic control, and finally focusing on improving health care behaviours, such as improving diet, increasing exercise, monitoring blood glucose (and, if hypertensive, monitor blood pressure with a home blood pressure device) and increasing other pleasurable activities.

## CONCLUSIONS

There is a high prevalence of depressive and anxiety disorders in patients with diabetes, and these disorders adversely affect diabetes self-care, disease control and clinical outcomes. Complications of diabetes resulting in functional impairment can also precipitate a depressive episode. Efficacy data have demonstrated that both evidence-based psychotherapies and pharmacotherapies are effective treatment modalities for depression in patients with diabetes. Collaborative care has been demonstrated to be an effective health service model to deliver high quality depression care to primary care populations with comorbid depression and diabetes. New models of collaborative care are also currently being tested to integrate depression care into TEAMcare approaches to diabetes care.

# REFERENCES

1. Anderson, R.J., Freedland, K.E., Clouse, R.E., and Lustman, P.J. (2001) The prevalence of comorbid depression in adults with diabetes: a meta-analysis. *Diabetes Care*, **24**, 1069–1078.
2. Ali, S., Stone, M.A., Peters, J.L. *et al.* (2006) The prevalence of co-morbid depression in adults with Type 2 diabetes: a systematic review and meta-analysis. *Diabet. Med.*, **23**, 1165–1173.
3. Ludman, E.J., Katon, W., Russo, J. *et al.* (2004) Depression and diabetes symptom burden. *Gen. Hosp. Psychiatry*, **26**, 430–436.
4. Von Korff, M., Katon, W., Lin, E.H. *et al.* (2005) Potentially modifiable factors associated with disability among people with diabetes. *Psychosom. Med.*, **67**, 233–240.
5. Simon, G., Katon, W., Lin, E. *et al.* (2005) Diabetes complications and depression as predictors of health care costs. *Gen. Hosp. Psychiatry*, **27**, 344–351.
6. Lin, E.H., Katon, W., Von Korff, M. *et al.* (2004) Relationship of depression and diabetes self-care, medication adherence, and preventive care. *Diabetes Care*, **27**, 2154–2160.
7. Katon, W., von Korff, M., Ciechanowski, P. *et al.* (2004) Behavioral and clinical factors associated with depression among individuals with diabetes. *Diabetes Care*, **27**, 914–920.
8. Katon, W.J., Lin, E.H., Russo, J. *et al.* (2004) Cardiac risk factors in patients with diabetes mellitus and major depression. *J. Gen. Intern. Med.*, **19**, 1192–1199.
9. Black, S.A., Markides, K.S., and Ray, L.A. (2003) Depression predicts increased incidence of adverse health outcomes in older Mexican Americans with type 2 diabetes. *Diabetes Care*, **26**, 2822–2828.
10. Katon, W.J., Rutter, C., Simon, G. *et al.* (2005) The association of comorbid depression with mortality in patients with type 2 diabetes. *Diabetes Care*, **28**, 2668–2672.
11. Katon, W., Fan, M.Y., Unutzer, J. *et al.* (2008) Depression and diabetes: a potentially lethal combination. *J. Gen. Intern. Med.*, **23**, 1571–1575.

12. Katon, W.J., Von Korff, M., Lin, E.H. *et al.* (2004) The Pathways Study: a randomized trial of collaborative care in patients with diabetes and depression. *Arch. Gen. Psychiatry*, **61**, 1042–1049.

13. Katon, W., Von Korff, M., Lin, E. *et al.* (1995) Collaborative management to achieve treatment guidelines. Impact on depression in primary care. *JAMA*, **273**, 1026–1031.

14. Licht-Strunk, E., Van Marwijk, H.W., Hoekstra, T. *et al.* (2009) Outcome of depression in later life in primary care: longitudinal cohort study with three years' follow-up. *BMJ*, **338**, a3079.

15. Vuorilehto, M.S., Melartin, T.K., and Isometsa, E.T. (2009) Course and outcome of depressive disorders in primary care: a prospective 18-month study. *Psychol. Med.*, **39**, 1697–1707.

16. Katon, W., Russo, J., Von Korff, M. *et al.* (2009) Depression and diabetes: factors associated with major depression at 5-year follow-up. *Psychosomatics*, **50**, 570–579.

17. Lustman, P.J., Griffith, L.S., Freedland, K.E., and Clouse, R.E. (1997) The course of major depression in diabetes. *Gen. Hosp. Psychiatry*, **19**, 138–143.

18. Alonso, J., Codony, M., Kovess, V. *et al.* (2007) Population level of unmet need for mental healthcare in Europe. *Br. J. Psychiatry*, **190**, 299–306.

19. Katon, W.J., Simon, G., Russo, J. *et al.* (2004) Quality of depression care in a population-based sample of patients with diabetes and major depression. *Med. Care*, **42**, 1222–1229.

20. Rush, A.J., Trivedi, M.H., Wisniewski, S.R. *et al.* (2006) Acute and longer-term outcomes in depressed outpatients requiring one or several treatment steps: a STAR*D report. *Am. J. Psychiatry*, **163**, 1905–1917.

21. Partnership for Solutions National Program Office (2001) Medicare 5% Standard Analytic File. Johns Hopkins University Press, Baltimore.

22. Petrak, F.and Herpertz, S. (2009) Treatment of depression in diabetes: an update. *Curr. Opin. Psychiatry*, **22**, 211–217.

23. van der Feltz-Cornelis, C., Nuyen, J., Stoop, C., *et al.* (2010) Effect of interventions for major depressive disorder and significant depressive symptoms in patients with diabetes mellitus: a systematic review and meta-analysis. *Gen. Hosp. Psychiatry*, doi: 10.1016/j.genhosppsych.2010.03.11.

24. Lustman, P.J., Griffith, L.S., Freedland, K.E. *et al.* (1998) Cognitive behavior therapy for depression in type 2 diabetes mellitus. A randomized, controlled trial. *Ann. Intern. Med.*, **129**, 613–621.

25. Huang, X., Song, L., Li, T. *et al.* (2002) Effect of health education and psychosocial intervention on depression in patients with type II diabetes. *Chin. Ment. Health J.*, **16**, 149–151.

26. Li, S., Li, M., Song, S. *et al.* (2003) The effect of psychological intervention in treating the diabetic patients with negative emotion. *Shandong J. Psychol. Med.*, **16**, 148.
27. Lu, S., Lu, B., and Gu, X. (2005) Cognitive therapy in combination with electromyographic feedback in treatment of diabetes patients with depression after cerebral infarction. *Chin. J. Clin. Pharm.*, **13**, 215–216.
28. Simson, U., Nawarotzky, U., Friese, G. *et al.* (2008) Psychotherapy intervention to reduce depressive symptoms in patients with diabetic foot syndrome. *Diabet. Med.*, **25**, 206–212.
29. Lustman, P.J., Griffith, L.S., Clouse, R.E. *et al.* (1997) Effects of nortriptyline on depression and glycemic control in diabetes: results of a double-blind, placebo-controlled trial. *Psychosom. Med.*, **59**, 241–250.
30. Lustman, P.J., Freedland, K.E., Griffith, L.S., and Clouse, R.E. (2000) Fluoxetine for depression in diabetes: a randomized double-blind placebo-controlled trial. *Diabetes Care*, **23**, 618–623.
31. Paile-Hyvarinen, M., Wahlbeck, K., and Eriksson, J.G. (2003) Quality of life and metabolic status in mildly depressed women with type 2 diabetes treated with paroxetine: a single-blind randomised placebo controlled trial. *BMC Fam. Pract.*, **4**, 7.
32. Xue, H. (2004) Paroxetine for depression in diabetes: a randomized controlled trial. *Chin. Ment. Health J.*, **18**, 735–737.
33. Gulseren, L., Gulseren, S., Hekimsoy, Z., and Mete, L. (2005) Comparison of fluoxetine and paroxetine in type II diabetes mellitus patients. *Arch. Med. Res.*, **36**, 156–165.
34. Paile-Hyvarinen, M., Wahlbeck, K., and Eriksson, J.G. (2007) Quality of life and metabolic status in mildly depressed patients with type 2 diabetes treated with paroxetine: a double-blind randomised placebo controlled 6-month trial. *BMC Fam. Pract.*, **8**, 34.
35. Hedges, L. and Olkin, I. (1985) *Statistical Methods for Meta-Analysis*, Academic Press, Orlando.
36. Lipsey, M.W. and Wilson, D.B. (1993) The efficacy of psychological, educational, and behavioral treatment. Confirmation from meta-analysis. *Am. Psychol.*, **48**, 1181–1209.
37. Katon, W.J. and Seelig, M. (2008) Population-based care of depression: team care approaches to improving outcomes. *J. Occup. Environ. Med.*, **50**, 459–467.
38. Kroenke, K., Spitzer, R., and Williams, J. (2001) The PHQ-9: validity of a brief depression severity measure. *J. Gen. Intern. Med.*, **16**, 606–613.
39. Meeuwissen, J.A., van der Feltz-Cornelis, C.M., van Marwijk, H.W. *et al.* (2008) A stepped care programme for depression management: an

uncontrolled pre-post study in primary and secondary care in The Netherlands. *Int. J. Integr. Care*, **8**, e05.

40. Gilbody, S., Bower, P., Fletcher, J. *et al.* (2006) Collaborative care for depression: a cumulative meta-analysis and review of longer-term outcomes. *Arch. Intern. Med.*, **166**, 2314–2321.

41. Williams, J.W. Jr., Katon, W., Lin, E.H. *et al.* (2004) The effectiveness of depression care management on diabetes-related outcomes in older patients. *Ann. Intern. Med.*, **140**, 1015–1024.

42. Ell, K., Katon, W., and Xie, B. (2010) Collaborative care management of major depression among low-income Hispanics with diabetes: a randomized controlled trial. *Diabetes Care*, **33**, 706–713.

43. Lin, E.H.B., Katon, W., Rutter, C. *et al.* (2006) Effects of enhanced depression treatment on diabetes self-care. *Ann. Fam. Med.*, **4**, 46–53.

44. Berkman, L.F., Blumenthal, J., Burg, M. *et al.* (2003) Effects of treating depression and low perceived social support on clinical events after myocardial infarction: the Enhancing Recovery in Coronary Heart Disease Patients (ENRICHD) randomized trial. *JAMA*, **289**, 3106–3116.

45. Glassman, A.H., O'Connor, C.M., Califf, R.M. *et al.* (2002) Sertraline treatment of major depression in patients with acute MI or unstable angina. *JAMA*, **288**, 701–709.

46. Katon, W., Unutzer, J., Fan, M.Y. *et al.* (2006) Cost-effectiveness and net benefit of enhanced treatment of depression for older adults with diabetes and depression. *Diabetes Care*, **29**, 265–270.

47. Simon, G.E., Katon, W.J., Lin, E.H. *et al.* (2007) Cost-effectiveness of systematic depression treatment among people with diabetes mellitus. *Arch. Gen. Psychiatry*, **64**, 65–72.

48. Katon, W.J., Russo, J.E., Von Korff, M. *et al.* (2008) Long-term effects on medical costs of improving depression outcomes in patients with depression and diabetes. *Diabetes Care*, **31**, 1155–1159.

49. Williams, M.M., Clouse, R.E., Nix, B.D. *et al.* (2007) Efficacy of sertraline in prevention of depression recurrence in older versus younger adults with diabetes. *Diabetes Care*, **30**, 801–806.

50. Lustman, P.J., Williams, M.M., Sayuk, G.S. *et al.* (2007) Factors influencing glycemic control in type 2 diabetes during acute- and maintenance-phase treatment of major depressive disorder with bupropion. *Diabetes Care*, **30**, 459–466.

51. Piette, J.D., Richardson, C., and Valenstein, M. (2004) Addressing the needs of patients with multiple chronic illnesses: the case of diabetes and depression. *Am. J. Manag. Care*, **10**, 152–162.

52. Teychenne, M., Ball, K., and Salmon, J. (2008) Physical activity and likelihood of depression in adults: a review. *Prev. Med.*, **46**, 397–411.

53. Horn, E.K., van Benthem, T.B., Hakkaart-van Roijen, L. *et al.* (2007) Cost-effectiveness of collaborative care for chronically ill patients with comorbid depressive disorder in the general hospital setting, a randomised controlled trial. *BMC Health Serv. Res.*, **7**, 28.
54. Katon, W. and Ciechanowski, P. (2009) Diabetes: psychosocial issues and psychiatric disorders, in *Comprehensive Texbook of Psychiatry* (eds M. Sadock, V. Sadock, and P. Ruiz), Lippincott, Williams and Wilkins, Philadelphia, PA, pp. 2294–2302.
55. Gilbody, S., Sheldon, T., and House, A. (2008) Screening and case-finding instruments for depression: a meta-analysis. *CMAJ*, **178**, 997–1003.
56. Gilbody, S.M., House, A.O., and Sheldon, T.A. (2001) Routinely administered questionnaires for depression and anxiety: systematic review. *BMJ*, **322**, 406–409.
57. Ludman, E., Katon, W., Russo, J. *et al.* (2006) Panic episodes among patients with diabetes. *Gen. Hosp. Psychiatry*, **28**, 475–481.
58. Trief, P.M., Ouimette, P., Wade, M. *et al.* (2006) Post-traumatic stress disorder and diabetes: co-morbidity and outcomes in a male veterans sample. *J. Behav. Med.*, **29**, 411–418.
59. Kroenke, K., Spitzer, R.L., Williams, J.B. *et al.* (2007) Anxiety disorders in primary care: prevalence, impairment, comorbidity, and detection. *Ann. Intern. Med.*, **146**, 317–325.
60. Morse, S.A., Ciechanowski, P.S., Katon, W.J., and Hirsch, I.B. (2006) Isn't this just bedtime snacking? The potential adverse effects of night-eating symptoms on treatment adherence and outcomes in patients with diabetes. *Diabetes Care*, **29**, 1800–1804.
61. American Diabetes Association (2007) Standards of medical care in diabetes. *Diabetes Care*, **30**, S4–S41.
62. Ijff, M., Huijbregts, K.M., van Marwijk, H.W. *et al.* (2007) Cost-effectiveness of collaborative care including PST and an antidepressant treatment algorithm for the treatment of major depressive disorder in primary care; a randomised clinical trial. *BMC Health Serv. Res.*, **7**, 34.
63. de Jong, F.J., van Steenbergen-Weijenburg, K.M., Huijbregts, K.M. *et al.* (2009) The Depression Initiative. Description of a collaborative care model for depression and of the factors influencing its implementation in the primary care setting in the Netherlands. *Int. J. Integr. Care*, **9**, e81.
64. Katon, W., Lin, E., Von Korff, M. *et al.* (2010) Integrating depression and chronic disease care among patients with diabetes and/or coronary heart disease: the design of the TEAMcare study. *Contemp. Clin. Trials*, **31**, 312–322.

# CHAPTER 5

# Diabetes and Depression: Management in Ordinary Clinical Conditions

**Richard Hellman**

*Department of Medicine, University of Missouri, Kansas City, MO, USA*

**Paul Ciechanowski**

*Department of Psychiatric and Behavioral Sciences, University of Washington School of Medicine, Seattle, WA, USA*

Effective treatment of depression in patients with diabetes often depends upon the success of their overall care. Yet, as most clinicians discover, the success of the overall care of patients with diabetes also depends upon the effective treatment of comorbid depression.

The interplay between the two conditions is even more complex when short- or long-term cognitive dysfunction complicates the care of both diabetes and depression. There is widespread agreement on the close relationship between diabetes, depression and cognitive dysfunction, as well as a general appreciation about how much each of these three conditions impacts patients' overall health and the course of their other chronic conditions. There is also evidence that the relationship between diabetes, depression and cognitive dysfunction is bidirectional, and that each condition may increase both the risk of and severity of each of the other conditions [1–6].

*Depression and Diabetes*   Edited by Wayne Katon, Mario Maj and Norman Sartorius
© 2010 John Wiley & Sons, Ltd

It is no surprise that the costs of care related to diabetes and depression are also greatly increased through the interaction of both conditions [7]. It is also known that when these conditions co-exist, there is greater risk for adverse clinical outcomes and increased mortality [8–11]. As an example, depression in a patient with diabetes is often more severe, prolonged and recurrent [12–14].

There is evidence that effective treatment of depression in patients with diabetes is urgently needed, and published data from a number of trials, using a variety of clinical approaches, show significant improvement in important parameters [15–23]. Nevertheless, the majority of patients with diabetes and depression, many of whom have cognitive dysfunction, remain undiagnosed and their depression remains untreated [24, 25]. Even those who are diagnosed often receive suboptimal care with disappointing results [26].

In this chapter, some of the most important barriers to delivering effective treatment for depression in individuals with diabetes are reviewed. Also explored are the complexities that potentially arise from hyperglycaemia, which worsens both depression and cognitive dysfunction and, in turn, is further associated with poorer glycaemic control and decreased efficacy of interventional efforts to deal with the depressed state of the patient [27]. How acute hypoglycaemia may potentially lead to accidents and worsen both depression and anxiety, affecting longer-term decisions, is discussed. The cultural and linguistic barriers that become important when treatment plans are implemented are described, highlighting some of the special problems noted in different countries and ethnic groups. Steps for optimizing patient–provider collaboration during the treatment of depression in patients with diabetes are discussed. How patients' experiences of concurrent diabetes and depression symptoms can lead to difficulties in recognition and diagnosis of depression in patients with diabetes is described. How depression in patients with diabetes may negatively influence treatment adherence, lead to emotional eating, significantly alter healthcare use patterns and undermine trust in the clinical relationship is reviewed, too. Appropriate clinical and psychoeducational approaches are also discussed.

Although the obstacles to optimal care of diabetes and depression are daunting, recent trial data and increased understanding of the complexities of care give us good reason to be optimistic about the future. In this chapter current changes in recommendations for care and promising multidisciplinary efforts now underway for the treatment of diabetes and depression are discussed.

## THE IMPACT OF SETTINGS ON THERAPY

The earlier seminal works of A. Kleinman and N. Sartorius have clearly delineated the profound ways in which culture affects the diagnosis and management of depression. Since the setting in which an individual lives and his/her culture play a profound role in each aspect of a person's life, it is no surprise that successful treatment strategies for those with diabetes and depression must be culturally sensitive as well. Even the recognition of depression and the diagnosis itself may be affected by the cultural beliefs, customs and mores of the particular social milieu, and, as a result, it is often difficult to establish the true incidence of depression in many countries.

In cultures where there has been a history of great hardships, such as in the People's Republic of China, there may be great difficulty distinguishing between sadness, which is viewed as common, a fact of life that needs to be accepted, and the clinical condition of depression, where the individual has symptoms of dysfunction, some of which may not be socially acceptable and may even be condemned [28]. There are many countries in which social stigma commonly accompanies the diagnosis of depression [29, 30]. In a setting where patients feel their symptoms of depression reflect badly upon them and upon their family, a diagnosis of depression will be harder to make, since denial is common, and in the place of symptoms commonly associated with major clinical depression, there may be primarily somatization (e.g. 'I feel dizzy') [28, 31]. In China, a recent study showed that the diagnosis of depression in those with heart disease is delayed, leading to more severe degrees of disability [32]. This is also a problem in other cultures as well [33–37]. For example, in a setting where fatalism is a common feature and an important part of the culture, attempts to treat depression may be resisted. In some Asian and Native American cultures, traditional beliefs may interfere with treatment of depression, both in terms of use of medication and how psychological therapies are viewed [38]. Fatalism, a belief that the outcome has already been pre-determined and attempts to alter the course are futile, may have a religious or cultural basis. But it is also common in many other settings and, in some cases, may be reinforced by the care provider. Physicians anxious to demonstrate their competence all too often try to predict the future course of the disease, and their prediction may be interpreted by the patient as what will certainly occur. Such a belief may inhibit the patient's own initiative in self-care and self-protective behaviours.

Also, in a number of cultures, strong beliefs in alternative therapies lead to preferences to use these therapies to treat both diabetes and depression. There is abundant literature that delineates the use of traditional Chinese medical practices, such as acupuncture, wearing brocade, herbal medicines and other alternative therapies. Moreover, in some Latino cultures, it is commonly believed that managing diabetes cannot be successful without assessing, managing and treating 'susto', defined as a state of anxiety or stress [39–42]. In this setting, clinical symptoms of depression may not be identified as a separate clinical condition. The symptoms associated with depression also may be different between cultures [43].

Language also presents barriers to care of the depressed patient with diabetes. Too often, the provider of care does not fully understand the language of the patient and important nuances of meaning are lost, further complicating the therapeutic intervention [44]. Translators, if not well trained, may be overconfident in their ability to correctly capture the meaning of either side of the two-way conversation, and, in some circumstances, may deliberately provide an incomplete or misleading translation [45].

A number of major patient advocacy groups, including Latino and Native American organizations, have raised concerns about the all too common practice of using family members as medical translators for the patient. They point out that often the content of the questions asked may lead to great embarrassment both to the family and to the patient, and thus alienation from and mistrust of the care providers. A better alternative is, whenever possible, to use a professional medical translator.

Fortunately, there are several effective solutions in dealing with language barriers in the treatment of depression. Several tools used to objectively diagnose depression and to evaluate its severity have been validated in different languages and in different countries [46, 47]. These may be particularly useful in providing a more objective evaluation and monitoring of the depressed patient [46–49]. Whenever there is a question or suspicion that there are significant barriers to communication, a qualified translator skilled in medical terminology should be used. Even then, it is necessary to be careful that the dialect of the language being used by the translator is fully comprehended by the patient. At the same time, determining whether an intermediary has to assist on the cultural context of the patient would also be helpful.

There are also useful tools for the diagnosis and evaluation of cognitive dysfunction, a comorbid condition where language, educational background and culture play an important role in the performance and validity of the tool [50]. Because of the importance of understanding the cultural and personal context, great care must be taken to respectfully and carefully obtain a family and personal history, in order to develop a model for the context needed for interpreting the symptoms of the patient.

Another crucial step for the healthcare provider is to understand how treatment of diabetes itself is seen through the prism of the patient's culture. Psychological distress may be related to demands of the care regimen, fears regarding the potential effects of the diabetes upon the future and the limitations that occur because of complications, disability or illness. Patients' fears and beliefs and the impact on their decisions may be profoundly shaped by cultural influences. For example, the effect of a fatalistic philosophy on a patient's response to a treatment plan of a diabetic foot ulcer is often to delay or not seek treatment at all, or to stop treatment after it has begun.

A recurring challenge in the treatment of depression in a patient with diabetes is the interplay between the physical challenges of diabetes and the emotional distress of depression, which requires coordination between groups of providers whose expertise does not overlap, who may not be part of the same clinical entity and who seldom communicate with each other on a timely basis [51]. This is why some of the most successful efforts in treating diabetes and depression have been structured to facilitate ready clinical exchange between a mental health professional, a primary care provider and, in some cases, a specialist providing diabetes care. While there are no trials that fully integrate the psychological services with the continuing care of the physical needs of patients with diabetes, such trials will likely be forthcoming. Resultant data from such efforts will be crucial as new models of care are developed for those with diabetes and depression.

In settings where the provider of healthcare is not well acquainted with the culture of the patient, or is not certain as to how the information is being received by the patient, it is very useful to ask more open-ended questions that encourage the patient to explain how the condition under discussion is understood or treated in his/her culture; for example, whether others in their family with a similar condition may have received traditional therapies. Of particular interest are the cultural beliefs, attitudes, traditional therapies and stigma associated with both diabetes and depression, but many important barriers of these types may become clearer as the therapeutic process unfolds, and resolve only as the patient–provider relationship strengthens.

When a cultural barrier is found, it is most important to identify it as an issue to be handled with respect. An example of this would be the stigma of depression in patients of Chinese ancestry. It may be helpful to acknowledge that the stigma to the diagnosis of depression is common and upsetting to the patient, but also to point out that more modern medicine and therapy can not only relieve the depression, and lead to a much better quality of life for the patient, but also lead to better family and community harmony as well. This strategy may encourage the patients to both actively participate in therapy for their depression, as well as help the clinician to motivate them to improve their diabetes care.

## THE CLINICAL INTERPLAY BETWEEN DEPRESSION, COGNITIVE DYSFUNCTION, DIABETIC COMPLICATIONS AND GLYCAEMIC CONTROL

One of the most important barriers to the successful treatment of depression in the patient with diabetes is the tight interrelationship between glycaemic control, cognitive status and mood [52, 53]. There is a biophysiologic basis for this relationship [54–57]. Put simply, if glucose control is suboptimal, it is likely to have an adverse effect upon the depression and cognitive dysfunction, and each, in turn, may complicate the efforts for glycaemic control [58, 59]. Moreover, if an accident or clinical adverse event occurs as a result of suboptimal glycaemic control and causes injury, morbidity or disability, that too will have an additive effect upon the burden of the depression.

For a number of years, there has been awareness that acute changes in glycaemic control can affect both cognition and mood [60, 61]. The careful studies of Cox and his colleagues have shown clearly that severe cognitive dysfunction occurs not only with glycaemic levels under 45 mg/dl (2.5 mmol/l), but also with acute hyperglycaemia over 325 mg/dl (18.0 mmol/l) [60]. He has further shown the vulnerability of the patient in driving simulators. These data, most importantly, indicate that judgment is one of the first aspects of cognitive function to be affected. Although the patients who were in a driving simulator gradually became aware that they were somewhat hypoglycaemic, they generally misjudged how severely affected they were, and incorrectly thought their performance was adequate while they were in the driving simulator, despite clear, objective evidence that they were very dysfunctional and would have been a danger to themselves or others if actually driving a motor vehicle [62].

The key point derived from such data is relevant because it shows that the choices the persons with diabetes make while either markedly hypoglycaemic or hyperglycaemic complicate their subsequent care and make them vulnerable to errors of self-medication (e.g. wrong medicine, wrong dose, wrong time, missed medication) [58]. These factors substantially increase the risk for poor outcomes and, in particular, worsen comorbid anxiety and depression, while also distracting them from effectively undertaking self-management tasks. Other data show that depression is associated with a delayed onset of care for diabetic foot ulcers, a delay that often leads to increased morbidity, and often to disability and earlier death [63, 64].

Patients with diabetes have a greatly increased incidence of cardiovascular disease [65]. The increased incidence varies from twofold to fourfold. In those patients with diabetes who smoke cigarettes, the total risk of cardiovascular events may be as high as 15 times that of a non-smoking person without diabetes, the highest relative risks being for peripheral vascular disease [66]. Additionally, for each cardiovascular event, patients with diabetes have a higher risk of morbidity and mortality than those without diabetes. But the correlation between cardiac events and death is even stronger for depression than it is for diabetes [67–69]. In other words, patients with diabetes who also have depression have a greatly increased cardiovascular risk, since depression and adverse cardiovascular events are very closely linked. Furthermore, independent of depression, diabetes also carries an increased vulnerability, not only because of the increased incidence of cardiovascular disease in diabetes, but also because of the patient's decreased awareness of chest pain and/or peripheral vascular pain as a result of diabetic neuropathy [70, 71]. In addition, many persons with diabetes have multiple comorbid conditions which may further increase the burden and risk of depression. As a general rule, multiple comorbid conditions are usually additive in their adverse effects on function and mood [71–74].

There are abundant data to show that cognitive dysfunction, a condition not often screened for in patients with diabetes, is much more common than usually thought, and has an independent adverse effect upon the patient's care. It should not come as a surprise to clinicians caring for individuals with diabetes that short-term and longer-term cognitive dysfunction both negatively impact patients' self-management routines [68, 75]. Experienced educators have long warned that education in self-management 'survival skills' often cannot be successfully taught just after an episode of diabetic ketoacidosis, severe hyperglycaemia, or severe hypoglycaemia, because of the impairment in memory and cognition that occurs after each of these events. However, contrary to popular belief, evidence linking severe, recurrent hypoglycaemia to long-term cognitive deficit is lacking, apart from those patients who were severely hypoglycaemic and under six years of age, a time of great vulnerability of the human brain. In fact, lower average blood glucose levels, as assessed by glycosylated haemoglobin levels, is associated with improved long-term cognition [76, 77].

Only recently has some of the biophysiologic basis for the longer-term adverse effect of hyperglycaemia on cognitive function been elucidated [55]. There is evidence that the prefrontal areas of the brain respond to hyperglycaemia with an increase in the levels of glutamate-glutamine-γ-aminobutyric acid, which is associated with objective evidence of both cognitive dysfunction and mild depression [56].

The finding is not surprising, since glutamate receptors play a very important role in memory.

In addition, insulin affects distinct cognitive processes by triggering the formation of psychological memory contents. There is evidence that insulin resistance in the brain may be a common denominator of cognitive dysfunction [55]. In patients with diabetes, cognitive function is not only adversely affected by both hypo- and hyperglycaemia, but also by the presence of acute cerebrovascular events. Cognitive function is also affected by inflammatory factors, which may begin a cascade of events that result in the increased intracerebral accumulation of amyloid [55]. The effect of inflammatory factors in the brain may be one of the important mechanisms by which central insulin resistance affects cognition. Other chronic vascular changes, common in diabetes, also affect cognition. Hyperactivity of the hypothalamic–pituitary–adrenal (HPA) axis may also potentially have negative effects on cognitive function in individuals with diabetes. For example, it is thought that chronically elevated levels of cortisol can lead to disorders of cognition, as well as depression [78]. Each of these mechanisms may be additive in its effects.

Some compelling data on the effect of cognitive dysfunction on clinical outcomes come from a recently reported multinational trial, the ADVANCE trial, which examined data from 11 140 patients from 215 centres in 20 countries. One arm of the trial evaluated the relationship between cognitive decline and how it affected the blood pressure and glycaemia lowering efforts in the trial [79]. The ADVANCE trial investigators used a Mini-Mental Status Exam (MMSE) score to stratify the patients into normal (MMSE score $\geq 28$), mild (MMSE 24–27) and severe cognitive dysfunction (MMSE $\leq 23$) and evaluated their outcomes. Both mild and severe cognitive dysfunction were associated with a significant increase in the adjusted rates of major cardiovascular events (HR 1.27, $p < 0.05$), cardiovascular death (HR 1.41, $p \leq 0.05$) and all-cause death (HR 1.33, $p < 0.03$). Severe, but not mild, cognitive dysfunction increased the risk of severe hypoglycaemia (HR 2.10, $p = 0.018$). But cognitive dysfunction did not ameliorate the beneficial effects of either blood pressure or glucose lowering in the risks of major cardiovascular events. It was concluded that, although chronic cognitive dysfunction is a major contributor to excess morbidity and mortality, and to the risk of major accident (severe hypoglycaemia), it is not a reason to withhold intensive glycaemic therapy.

This important study shows that cognitive dysfunction is an independent risk factor for the patient with diabetes, but there are other data that show the close linkage between cognitive dysfunction and depression. Cognitive dysfunction increases the risk for depression [24]. And depression in diabetes is associated with poorer glycaemic control, which in turn is associated with both an increased frequency and severity of depression and cognitive dysfunction [24, 59, 60]. A recent study has shown that comorbid depression in adult patients with diabetes increased the risk of development of dementia by 2.7-fold over a five-year period [80].

There is a misconception that cognitive dysfunction is a disorder primarily affecting those over 65 years of age. Clearly, in patients with diabetes, this is not the case. Acute cognitive dysfunction may occur at any age and at any time in those with diabetes, if their glycaemic control is sufficiently poor. There is evidence that cognitive dysfunction that is permanent can occur from long-term hyperglycaemia, even in young individuals with diabetes [81]. A child or adolescent who cannot keep up with his peers is subject to severe emotional distress and the mutually reinforcing problems noted contribute greatly to the complexity of his care.

Cognitive dysfunction in the patient with diabetes may be reversible if the underlying cause can be reversed or treated. Examples of these are well known, including improved glycaemic control and avoidance of severe hypo- or hyperglycaemia. Improvement in blood pressure control is another example of a treatable condition that may lead to improvement in cognitive function. In some cases, the correction of severe chronic renal failure, improvement of cerebral blood flow or reduction of overmedication may result in significant cognitive improvement. Depression may occur as a secondary reaction to the onset of cognitive function and worsen the memory and concentration problems. Treatment of comorbid depression may improve cognitive function. But all too often, chronic cognitive dysfunction in a patient with diabetes, which often occurs well before the age of 65, may not have an effective remedy, in contrast to depression, for which there are effective psychological therapies and medications. In this case, cognitive dysfunction needs to be considered as a confounder, a barrier to the therapy for diabetes care and the care of depression. As in the case of the depression therapy, the interdependent comorbid condition of chronic cognitive dysfunction needs to be identified and accounted for if the therapy for overall diabetes care and for depression is to be successful.

Coordination of care of the person with diabetes is a difficult task, made much more challenging by the presence of depression or cognitive dysfunction, or both [5, 82]. Errors in care may occur by the patient, their family, or their care providers, because of key information that may be known by only one of the parties, which is not transmitted in a timely fashion to the other providers or to the patient.

This lack of collaboration between the providers diminishes each of their efforts and hampers the all-important collaboration with the patient. In different locales the healthcare structure, the culture, the economics and the workforce will greatly influence what is possible regarding coordination, collaboration and information sharing. But as long as each of the care providers is aware of some of the common pitfalls of not coordinating the care of the patient with diabetes and depression, their efforts may be more likely to be successful in ordinary clinical settings.

The initial assessment and review of the patient should be as complete as possible. All patients with diabetes should initially be given a screening questionnaire for depression that is culturally appropriate and in their language. However, there are no data that show the advantage of one depression screening tool over all others [83–86]. The initial screen may uncover many patients who may have the diagnosis of depression but have not volunteered clinical symptoms. But the diagnosis of major depression must be validated by an experienced clinician, a crucial step necessary to avoid overdiagnosis and overtreatment. The current screening instruments for depression generally demonstrate sensitivity of 80–90% and specificity of 70–85% [86]. Several researchers have estimated that 24–47% of positive screens will meet specific criteria for major depressive disorder. This point needs to be emphasized. More than half of the positive results for depression obtained by the most commonly used screening tools will not prove to indicate a major depression; instead, the patient may be found to have either a milder form of depression- or diabetes-related psychological distress, or another diagnostic entity altogether [87].

The optimal intervention for screening for depression has not been established, but expert clinical opinion supports using a regular interval to review, at least yearly, the relative risk factors for depression of the patient in order to determine the need for screening for depression and subsequent verification of major depressive disorder by DSM-IV criteria [84].

It is important to understand that there is no evidence that screening for depression followed by feedback to the provider alone will result in better outcomes for the patient [84]. Evidence of benefit has occurred when screening for depression is associated with coordinated efforts to provide a structured programme for those patients with depression [84].

Testing for cognitive dysfunction can be justified because both short-term and long-term cognitive dysfunction may exist in all age groups. Unfortunately, no single test is both necessary and sufficient. The 'gold standard', a careful and complete cognitive evaluation of cognitive dysfunction, can be done by a qualified neuropsychologist, but this is both time consuming, resource intensive and expensive, and is usually not routinely available.

In general, there is a dearth of data on culturally and linguistically sensitive tools for cognitive dysfunction. There are some on-line tools [88] that rely heavily upon cognitive testing that is less dependent upon language and educational level, but there are not sufficient data to establish them as a standard. Initially, age-appropriate, linguistically and culturally appropriate tools should be used to test for cognitive dysfunction, during any clinical scenario when there is a reasonable expectation that cognitive dysfunction should be important.

Since short-term cognitive dysfunction may be the result of rapidly correctable problems, such as severe hypoglycaemia or severe hyperglycaemia, the cognitive test chosen should help to identify the short-term problem, and allow the clinician to convince either the patient or the family that cognitive dysfunction is present. Then the clinician may check the patient's glucose level, verify the level of glucose and begin treatment aimed at returning the glucose to more normal levels. This, however, may not immediately correct the cognitive dysfunction. For example, if a person has a glucose level of <45 mg% (2.5 mmol/l), even when fully corrected it may take at least 45 minutes before their judgment is sufficient to allow for safe driving of a motor vehicle [89].

Testing for cognitive dysfunction, however, should be done not only initially but repeated as the need arises. For example, it is crucial to demonstrate to the patient that while he/she is hypoglycaemic, his/her acute functioning would make driving a vehicle unsafe. When interpreting cognitive function testing, it is critically important to be aware of the present glycaemic levels and their recent control. Evidence of other chronic diseases, such as advanced renal failure, will also increase the risk for cognitive dysfunction.

The presence of cognitive dysfunction as measured objectively should be documented. If there is a reversible cause, the problem should be corrected and the patient retested, but if the problem is not correctable, for example, chronic renal failure or cerebrovascular disease, the therapy plan and education plan should be altered to increase patient levels of safety.

## COORDINATION OF CARE AND USE OF TREATMENTS FOR DEPRESSION

Transfer of information between providers should be timely, patient centred and continuous. The mental health provider performance will be improved by their added knowledge. For adults without staff-assisted depression supports in place, there is a reasonable certainty that the net benefit of screening is small [84]. In contrast, with such supports in place, there is a reasonable certainty that the benefit of screening is at least moderate [83]. The recent US Preventative Services Task Force review of this subject found good evidence to support this conclusion [90]. Therefore, it is recommended that the practice setting should be modified so that both the diabetes care and the depression treatment allow for the special needs of the patient with diabetes and depression. Core supports may include a nurse care manager, institutional commitment to train with the aid of workshops, monthly lectures, staff and clinician training, and phone support. But it is also important that the primary care clinician or specialist treating the diabetes be aware of the progress of the patient and involved in the team approach.

It is recommended that the mental health clinician should coordinate with primary care physicians and avoid medications for depression that have a high risk for side effects to which the person with diabetes may be particularly sensitive. Amitriptyline, desipramine and nortriptyline are associated with relatively high incidence of cardiac and cardiovascular side effects, including arrhythmias and orthostatic hypotension as well as hyperglycemia.

In addition, with the use of antidepressants, there is an increased risk of the serotonin syndrome, also called serotonin toxicity, a rare but potentially lethal syndrome, characterized by cognitive, autonomic and somatic effects due to an increase in 5-HT levels in the central nervous system. Originally found with monoamine oxidase (MAO) inhibitors, serotonin syndrome has been found with selective serotonin reuptake inhibitors (SSRIs), tricyclic antidepressants, bupropion, St. John's wort and many other drugs. Drug interactions are a common precipitating event [91].

There is no conclusive evidence, either from the US Preventative Services Task Force [84] or the STAR*D trial [92], that one antidepressant medication is superior to all of the others. Many patients will fail to respond to the initial choice of antidepressant. Failure to continue the medication is frequent: 16–29% of treatments with SSRIs are discontinued for any reason within the first two months [93]. Sixty-one percent of all patients on SSRIs have at least one side effect (e.g. nausea, headaches, diarrhoea, fatigue, dizziness, sexual dysfunction), but the reasons for discontinuation may vary widely and may not be related to side effects [87]. Often the tolerability profile of one medication may not be optimal for the particular patient.

The risk for suicide for a patient on antidepressants is very small, and for older patients on antidepressant medication there is a marked reduction in suicidal behaviours. The risk factors for increased rate of suicide or self-harm include comorbid alcohol use, history of self-harm, use of antipsychotic medication, a mental health referral (most likely a proxy for more serious disorders) and the use of more than one antidepressant [87].

Regarding completed suicides, none of several meta-analyses of short-term trials of adults treated for major depressive disorder supplied clear evidence that any second-generation antidepressant significantly increased the rates of completed suicide as compared with placebo. In contrast, the highest odds of non-fatal suicidal behaviour in adults for all ages was reported when major depressive disorder was treated with paroxetine (odds ratio 6.70; CI: 1.1, 149.4), with most events occurring in those aged 18–29 years. Suicide attempts are highest in those under 18 [84, 87].

St. John's wort is to be avoided because of the lack of demonstrated efficacy in depression and the multiple significant drug interactions, particularly with anticoagulants, that occur. Preparations of St. John's wort induce the liver cytochrome P-450 enzymes, particularly CYP3A4 and also CYP2C9. This will increase the metabolism and decrease the efficacy of many drugs [94].

There is a risk of gastrointestinal bleeding in older adults in patients on antidepressants [95–97], particularly in those on SSRIs, with an excess risk of 3.1 bleeds/1000 patient years in a Danish study [97]. A Canadian study showed that patients over age 65 years taking non-steroidal anti-inflammatory drugs in addition to an antidepressant had an even higher risk, with a relative risk of 2.8 [95].

In another study in patients aged 50 years or older, SSRI use was associated with an increased risk of fragility fractures (hazard ratio 2.1; CI: 1.3, 3.4), as well as a twofold increased risk of falls [98]. It is recommended that antidepressants be considered cautiously, as they place the elderly or frail person with diabetes at significantly higher risk for falls, and the care support should be adjusted appropriately. In general, however, the SSRIs are well tolerated by most patients. Discontinuation in older patients due to side effects ranged from 17 to 22%, and overall discontinuation from 32 to 36% within three months [87].

The choice of antidepressant medication for the patient with diabetes and depression remains one in which the clinician needs to individualize therapy to the specific needs of the patient. There are strong data showing that the specific initial choice of antidepressant, with the aforementioned exceptions, may be less crucial than the duration of appropriate therapy, the coordination of psychiatric and medical care, and the input of the clinician in modification of dose or choice of medication dependent upon the response to therapy. The patient's tolerance to a specific antidepressant is not predictable, in part due to genetic variations in the metabolism of specific medications, as well as other less well studied aspects of biologic variability.

One caveat worth noting is the onset of new symptoms. The presence, for example, of unexpected hyperactivity, insomnia and agitation may be a reflection of a bipolar mood disorder and the mental health provider should be contacted for an alternative medication plan.

There is now strong scientific evidence that depressive symptoms in persons with diabetes can be successfully treated with both psychotherapeutic techniques, such as cognitive behavioural therapy, and antidepressant drugs, but there is little evidence that it is possible to improve either glycaemic control or mortality or reduce complications with successful depression treatments [84].

There is one randomized controlled trial, the Prospect Trial, which noted reduction of death rates in the diabetes subset of patients who were treated with a well-coordinated depression programme which used a trained nurse manager to facilitate care [15], but subset analyses are often misleading, and the study results have not gained wide acceptance.

The Pathways and IMPACT studies have clearly shown the cost benefits of a coordinated depression management programme, but more data are needed [7, 16]. It is likely that longer-term programmes which tightly integrate mental health efforts with the diabetes control and overall management are more likely to show not only improvement of depression, but also improved clinical diabetes outcomes. The development of further appropriately structured and powered trials is eagerly looked forward to.

## OPTIMIZING THE PROVIDER–PATIENT RELATIONSHIP

Clinical depression is characterized by a constellation of cognitive (e.g. impaired concentration), emotional (e.g. sad mood) and somatic (e.g. fatigue) symptoms. Irrespective of specific diagnosis (e.g. major or minor depression), there is a limited subset of symptoms that individuals experience when they are depressed. According to the DSM-IV, patients with major or minor depression must exhibit either depressed mood and/or significant loss of pleasure for at least a two-week period. However, other salient depressive symptoms include fatigue, lack of concentration, increased or decreased appetite, insomnia or hypersomnia, or feeling agitated or slowed down. Each of these depressive symptoms mimics symptoms that may be commonly experienced by patients with diabetes during the course of their illness. With excursions of blood glucose, for instance, fatigue, difficulty concentrating, changes in appetite, excessive sleepiness, or feelings of agitation or sluggishness can occur.

Over the past two decades, multiple studies [82, 99, 100] have also shown that depression amplifies diabetes symptoms, such as polyuria, polydipsia, hunger, shakiness, blurry vision and fatigue. In fact, individuals with depression are more likely to report diabetes symptoms, even after accounting for glucose levels as measured by glycosylated haemoglobin and the number of diabetes complications. The magnitude of this effect can be quite significant, with depressed diabetes patients being fourfold more likely to describe pain and numbness in their extremities, feeling faint or daytime sleepiness [82].

Whether they find it challenging to disentangle diabetes from depressive symptoms, or their diabetes symptoms are experienced to a greater degree because of concomitant depression, the individuals with comorbid depression and diabetes often experience frustration, confusion, hopelessness, or shame about not being able to control diabetes. Clinicians who understand the interplay between diabetes and depressive symptoms are in a strong position to make a difference by uncovering underlying depression when it exists, even when the patient's explanatory model focuses on diabetes as the cause of all symptoms.

Clinicians can augment their diagnostic skills in such cases through use of validated depression screening tools, such as the Patient Health Questionnaire – 9 (PHQ-9) [101], which can be completed by the patient in 1–2 minutes. To better assess stressors associated with or precipitating depression that are specifically related to diabetes, the clinician may benefit from using the Diabetes Distress Scale (DDS) [102], which examines stressful events ranging from minor hassles to major life difficulties in four domains: emotional burden, physician-related distress, regimen-related distress and interpersonal distress. The DDS is a valid measure that has been found to be associated with behavioural disease management variables and glycaemic control. In considering a diagnosis of depression in patients with diabetes, clinicians may also want to ask about risk factors for depression, including a history of depression or anxiety, mental health treatment, substance abuse or smoking, high medical comorbidity or presence of diabetes complications, or family history of depression or mental health treatment.

During the healthcare visit, there is a window of opportunity not only to make an accurate diagnosis of comorbid depression but also to educate the individual about what clinical events and mechanisms lie behind the experiences he/she is having. It can be quite relieving and comforting for the patient to finally understand that the symptoms he/she is living with may be primarily driven by depression. Clinically addressing these symptoms can begin to restore hope in a demoralized individual and help to forge a stronger therapeutic alliance. A psychoeducational approach is useful, where symptoms of depression and diabetes are reviewed and understood as having an overlap. Also pointing out to the patient that depression is commonly experienced as a physical symptom 'amplifier' can help the patient understand any recent failures in regaining stability of diabetic control and symptoms while depressed. Clinicians may also want to cite several research studies which showed that depression was a better predictor of diabetes symptoms than glycosylated haemoglobin or diabetes complications [82, 99].

Since over 95% of diabetes management is carried out by the patient [103], comorbid depression in diabetes commonly leads to lower adherence in carrying out day-to-day diabetes tasks, such as glucose monitoring, exercise, diet, and medication regimens. For example, in over 4000 patients with type 2 diabetes, Lin *et al.* [83] have shown that major depression was associated with less physical activity, unhealthy diet and, based on pharmacy refill data, lower adherence to oral hypoglycaemic, antihypertensive and lipid-lowering medications. Other studies have shown similar findings [104, 105]. Lack of motivation, poorer concentration, increased isolation, decreased ability to collaborate with others, fatigue and other associated symptoms of depression can all mediate this effect. Such behavioural lapses in self-care as well as central mechanisms related to the HPA axis and other neurophysiologic mechanisms may lead to glucose dyscontrol. Indeed, in a meta-analytic review of the literature, Lustman *et al.* [59] found a small to moderate, but significant, association between depression and hyperglycaemia in patients with type 1 and type 2 diabetes.

Depressive symptoms often smoulder for some time before they are identified and the associated lack of adherence, self-care and ability to successfully manage diabetes may lead to despondence and a sense of giving up in the patient, even before he/she is diagnosed as being depressed. By the time they are seen by a healthcare provider, patients may be resigned to believing they are unable to control their lifestyle and adequately control their diabetes whether they realize they are depressed or not. During the interaction with the healthcare provider, the patient may feel shame or embarrassment about his/her inability to better manage diabetes, especially if this is a relatively acute change for the person. Often there is a disconnect between the patient's rational ability to talk about what needs to take place to achieve glucose control and actual behaviours and action based on emotions. A prototypical statement by a depressed person in this situation may be: 'I know what I am supposed to do and what I am not supposed to do, but I still do the wrong things and I don't know why'. Clinicians, particularly when unaware of the patient's comorbid depression, may also feel discouraged given the recent lack of progress in disease status and may unwittingly blame the patient for not trying hard enough, which perpetuates self-negative cognitions the patient may have. It is helpful for the clinician to assume there is going to be a drop off in ability to self-manage diabetes during even a mild to moderate course of depression, and to expect that, if there is a relatively sudden decrease in level of self-management in a patient with diabetes, depression may be lurking.

Potentially exacerbating non-adherence issues in individuals with diabetes and comorbid depression is the commonplace use of food to regulate strong negative emotions. Eating disorders, such as binge eating, bulimia and subthreshold eating disorders, have been shown to be more prevalent among patients with type 1 and 2 diabetes than among medical control subjects [106–108] and can have significant negative consequences, including poorer dietary and glucose control and a greater likelihood of diabetes complications [109]. A potentially clinically significant and prevalent form of eating disorder among patients with diabetes is an eating pattern called night-eating syndrome, a syndrome closely tied to depression and emotional regulation. Among 714 tertiary care patients with type 1 and 2 diabetes, 10% reported night eating patterns in which >25% of their daily food intake was after regular suppertime [110]. Individuals engaging in night eating were more than twice as likely to have depression and reported eating in response to anger, sadness, loneliness, worry and being upset. Patients with night-eating behaviours were also over twice as likely to be obese, to have glycosylated haemoglobin values >7% and to have two or more diabetes complications.

Individuals with diabetes and underlying depression are also more likely to smoke cigarettes and have difficulty quitting smoking. In general, depression is twice as common in smokers than in non-smokers, and smokers with a lifetime history of depression are half as likely to quit smoking as compared to non-smokers [111, 112]. One cross-sectional survey of 183 smokers with diabetes and depression found a correlation between the number of cigarettes smoked and level of depression [113]. As with emotional eating, depressed patients may deem smoking helpful in regulating emotions and anxiety. The challenge for the healthcare provider in such circumstances is to maintain a non-judgmental stance, particularly around behaviour that carries a stigma, such as smoking and overeating, while providing effective support in changing behaviours once depressive symptoms begin to wane.

## HEALTH CARE USE

One of the first ways that a clinician may become aware that a patient is depressed is by observing changes in patterns of healthcare use. Patients may start making more appointments, calling more, or using urgent care or emergency services to a greater degree. On the other hand, patients may also begin to miss or cancel appointments. Studies have demonstrated that depression is associated with perturbations in healthcare use in both directions. For example, primary care use and costs have been shown to significantly increase in depressed individuals with diabetes. A study of 367 primary care patients showed that total healthcare costs were 86% higher for those with high depression severity compared to those with low severity [114]. Using data from the 1996 nationally representative Medical Expenditure Panel Survey, Egede *et al.* [115] reported that healthcare costs were 4.5 times as high in depressed patients as among those who were not depressed. Among 4398 adults with diabetes attending a health maintenance organization (HMO), after controlling for sociodemographic factors and duration and severity of diabetes, total healthcare costs were approximately 70% higher among those with major depression compared to those not depressed ($5361 vs $3120 six-month costs, $p < 0.001$) [7].

Depression has also been found to be associated with a significantly higher number of missed healthcare visits as measured by administrative data in patients with diabetes. In a study of 3900 patients with diabetes, those with major depression missed over twice as many scheduled and same day primary care appointments ($p < 0.001$ for both), as compared to those without depression [116]. In patients with diabetes, missed appointments have been associated with poorer glycaemic control [117, 118], lower glucose self-monitoring rates, non-adherence to oral hypoglycaemic medications [118], greater obesity levels, higher blood pressure, more microvascular complications [119] and lower rates of complication screening [119, 120]. There are many existing patient, organizational and provider level interventions designed to decrease missed appointments [121]. Clinicians may benefit from use of automated tracking of appointments, increased communication through telephone calls, e-mail and other web-based communication and use of proactive contacts such as mailed or telephoned reminders of appointments. By understanding how depressive symptoms lead to lack of motivation, poor concentration and difficulty with ability to organize one's life, providers and staff may achieve greater empathy and less frustration with their patients who miss appointments, while at the same time guiding patients toward more constructive healthcare use patterns.

Finally, clinicians should recognize that depression is associated with lower satisfaction with care [16] and with lower levels of trust [122]. However, with treatment of depression, trust and collaboration can improve. In a 10-month study in primary care patients with type 2 diabetes, it was shown that those patients whose depression decreased in severity over time had an increase in their ability to trust others, based on a measure of relationship style, as compared with patients in whom depression severity either did not change or worsened [122].

## CONCLUSIONS

There are many issues commonly encountered in day-to-day practice, including important clinical barriers, which are important to those treating patients with diabetes and depression.

Discussed has been the myriad of ways in which culture, country, language and custom may alter the presentation of those with diabetes and depression, the criteria for diagnosis, and factors that play a large role in the therapy offered and how it must be optimized.

The interplay between cognitive dysfunction, depression and diabetes has been discussed. Reviewed have been the ubiquitous presence of short-term cognitive dysfunction in diabetes care, and why and when longer-term cognitive dysfunction occurs, and the interaction between the risk factors, treatment of the depression, and the overall care of the patient. Also discussed has been the interaction between glycaemic control, cognition and mood, and it has been shown why cognitive dysfunction, as is depression, is so often associated with accidents in care and poor and unrealistic judgments. The issue of coordination of care has been discussed and why failure to coordinate key information between care providers and patients can lead to poorer outcomes.

Optimizing collaboration between the providers and depressed patients is crucial, since there is an association between ineffective provider–patient collaboration that results in lower levels of trust, poor information exchange and decreased satisfaction. The increased resistance of the patient that may develop may lead to both poorer adherence and poorer clinical outcomes [116]. Recent research exploring how patient relationship styles based on attachment theory may impact treatment adherence and diabetes outcomes may be relevant in clinical settings [123], particularly in working with patients who are depressed [122].

Each of the factors discussed in this chapter, the cultural barriers, the interplay between comorbid conditions and the strategies that foster strong patient–provider interchanges, is essential, since patients are often confused, demoralized and stressed by their fears of the future [124]. It is hoped that the understanding of the complexities of care and the need to enhance collaboration with a provider will lead to increased efforts to coordinate care. It is thought that, ideally, each patient with diabetes and depression would benefit from a multidisciplinary web of providers, so key clinical information is not lost, but instead can be used to best advantage for the patient during the therapy of both diabetes and depression [125–127].

The effect of depression on the treatment plan for diabetes is profound and complex. Because depression affects the ability of the patient to carry out his/her own plan of care, decreasing both the healthy lifestyle activities and the self-monitoring and medication usage, the clinician needs to be sure that depression is being effectively treated. More frequent telephone calls, better follow-up and a more understanding approach to how the depression may discourage and distract the patient is central to an effective treatment plan for those with diabetes and depression. The common occurrence of both short- and long-term cognitive dysfunction in the depressed diabetic patient also adds to the complexity of care and cost of care.

Since depressed patients with diabetes more often have an increased severity and high rate of recurrence of the depression, the mental health provider often will find that the medication course is more prolonged and the use of behavioural therapies is more crucial.

Successful management of diabetes and depression requires not only intensification of efforts in the therapy of depression as well as in medical therapy of diabetes, but a much higher level of prolonged cooperation between different disciplines for optimal results for the patient. Despite the evidence that the treatment for diabetes and depression is complex and more demanding than the treatment of either condition alone, published successful trials show that a well-coordinated plan of care is effective in treating these concurrent conditions.

## REFERENCES

1. Golden, S.H., Lazo, M., Carnethon, M. *et al.* (2008) Examining a bidirectional association between depressive symptoms and diabetes. *JAMA*, **299**, 2751–2759.
2. Mezuk, B., Eaton, W.W., Albrecht, S., and Golden, S.H. (2008) Depression and type 2 diabetes over the lifespan. *Diabetes Care*, **31**, 2383–2390.
3. Moussavi, S., Chatterji, S., Verdes, E. *et al.* (2007) Depression, chronic diseases, and decrements in health: results from the World Health Surveys. *Lancet*, **370**, 851–858.
4. Jaser, S.S., Holl, M.G., Jefferson, V., and Grey, M. (2009) Correlates of depressive symptoms in urban youth at risk for type 2 diabetes mellitus. *J. Sch. Health*, **79**, 286–292.
5. de Groot, M., Anderson, R., Freedland, K.E. *et al.* (2001) Association of depression and diabetes complication: a meta-analysis. *Psychosom. Med.*, **63**, 619–630.
6. Katon, W. (2003) Clinical and health services relationships between major depression, depressive symptoms, and general medical illness. *Biol. Psychiatry*, **54**, 216–226.
7. Simon, G.E., Katon, W.J., Lin, E.H.B. *et al.* (2005) Diabetes complications and depression as predictors of health service costs. *Gen. Hosp. Psychiatry*, **27**, 344–351.
8. Katon, W., Fan, M.Y., Unützer, J. *et al.* (2008) Depression and diabetes: a potentially lethal combination. *J. Gen. Intern. Med.*, **23**, 1571–1575.
9. Egede, L.E. (2004) Diabetes, major depression, and functional disability among U.S. adults. *Diabetes Care*, **27**, 421–428.
10. Von Korff, M., Katon, W., Lin, E.H.B. *et al.* (2005) Potentially modifiable factors associated with disability among people with diabetes. *Psychosom. Med.*, **67**, 233–240.
11. Egede, L.E., Nietert, P.J., and Zheng, D. (2005) Depression and all-cause and coronary heart disease mortality among adults with and without diabetes. *Diabetes Care*, **28**, 1339–1345.
12. Lustman, P.J., Griffith, L.S., and Clouse, R.E. (1988) Depression in adults with diabetes. Results of 5-yr follow-up study. *Diabetes Care*, **11**, 605–612.
13. Peyrot, M. and Rubin, R.R. (1999) Persistence of depressive symptoms in diabetic adults. *Diabetes Care*, **22**, 448–452.
14. Eaton, W., Shao, H., Nestadt, G. *et al.* (2008) Population-based study of first onset and chronicity in major depressive disorder. *Arch. Gen. Psychiatry*, **65**, 513–520.

15. Bogner, H.R., Morales, K.H., Post, E.P., and Bruce, J.L. (2007) Diabetes, depression, and death. *Diabetes Care*, **30**, 3005–3010.
16. Katon, W.J., Von Korff, M., Lin, E.H.B. *et al.* (2004) The Pathways study. *Arch. Gen. Psychiatry*, **61**, 1042–1049.
17. Katon, W.J., Russo, J.E., Von Korff, M. *et al.* (2008) Long-term effects on medical costs of improving depression outcomes in patients with depression and diabetes. *Diabetes Care*, **31**, 1155–1159.
18. Lustman, P.J., Griffith, L.S., Freedland, K.E. *et al.* (1998) Cognitive behavior therapy for depression in type 2 diabetes mellitus. *Ann. Intern. Med.*, **129**, 613–621.
19. Lustman, P.J., Williams, M.M., Sayuk, G.S. *et al.* (2007) Factors influencing glycemic control in type 2 diabetes during acute- and maintenance-phase treatment of major depressive disorder with bupropion. *Diabetes Care*, **30**, 459–466.
20. Lustman, P.J., Clouse, R.E., Nix, B.D. *et al.* (2006) Sertraline for prevention of depressive recurrence in diabetes mellitus. *Arch. Gen. Psychiatry*, **63**, 521–529.
21. Snoek, F.J., van der Ven, N.C.W., Twish, J.W.R. *et al.* (2008) Cognitive behavioural therapy (CBT) compared with blood glucose awareness training (BGAT) in poorly controlled Type 1 patient with diabetes: long-term effects on HbA1c moderated by depression. *Diabet. Med.*, **25**, 1337–1342.
22. Pouwer, F., Beekman, A.T.F., Lubach, C., and Snoek, F.J. (2006) Nurses' recognition and registration of depression, anxiety and diabetes-specific emotional problems in outpatients with diabetes mellitus. *Patient Educ. Couns.*, **60**, 235–240.
23. van Bastelaar, K.M.P., Pouwer, F., Cuijpers, P. *et al.* (2008) Web-based cognitive behavioural therapy (W-CBT) for diabetes patients with co-morbid depression: design of a randomised controlled trial. *BMC Psychiatry*, **8**, 9.
24. Munshi, M., Grande, L., Hayes, M. *et al.* (2006) Cognitive dysfunction is associated with poor diabetes control in older adults. *Diabetes Care*, **29**, 1797–1799.
25. de Wit, M., Delemarre-Van de Waal, H.A., Bokma, J.A. *et al.* Follow-up results on monitoring and discussing health-related quality of life in adolescent diabetes care: benefits do not sustain in routine practice. *Pediatric Diabetes* (in press).
26. Goldney, R.D., Phillips, P.J., Fisher, L.J., and Wilson, D.H. (2004) Diabetes, depression, and quality of life. *Diabetes Care*, **27**, 1066–1070.

27. Gonzalez, J.S., Peyrot, M., McCarl, L.A. *et al.* (2008) Depression and diabetes treatment nonadherence: a meta-analysis. *Diabetes Care*, **31**, 2398–2403.

28. Kleinman, A. (2004) Culture and depression. *N. Engl. J. Med.*, **351**, 951–953.

29. Hsu, L.K., Wan, Y.M., Chang, H. *et al.* (2008) Stigma of depression is more severe in Chinese Americans than Caucasian Americans. *Psychiatry*, **71**, 210–218.

30. Fogel, J. and Ford, D.E. (2005) Stigma beliefs of Asian Americans with depression in an internet sample. *Can. J. Psychiatry*, **50**, 470–478.

31. Hsu, L.K. and Folsten, M.F. (1997) Somatoform disorders in Caucasian and Chinese Americans. *J. Nerv. Ment. Dis.*, **185**, 382–387.

32. Teo, K.K., Lui, L., Chow, C.K. *et al.* (2009) Potentially modifiable risk factors associated with myocardial infarction in China: the INTERHEART China Study. *Heart*, **95**, 1857–1864.

33. Black, S.A., Markides, K.S., and Ray, L.A. (2003) Depression predicts increased incidence of adverse health outcomes in older Mexican Americans with type 2 diabetes. *Diabetes Care*, **26**, 2822–2828.

34. Papathanasiou, A., Shea, S., Koutsovasilis, A. *et al.* (2008) Reporting distress and quality of life of patients with diabetes mellitus in primary and secondary care in Greece. *Ment. Health Fam. Med.*, **5**, 85–93.

35. Takasaki, Y., Kawakami, N., Tsuchiya, M. *et al.* (2008) Heart disease, other circulatory diseases, and onset of major depression among community residents in Japan: results of the World Mental Health Survey Japan 2002–2004. *Acta Med. Okayama*, **62**, 241–249.

36. Lin, E.H.B. and Von Korff, M. on behalf of the WHO WMH Survey Consortium (2008) Mental disorders among persons with diabetes – results from the World Mental Health Survey. *J. Psychosom. Res.*, **65**, 571–580.

37. Zahid, N., Asghar, S., Claussen, B., and Hussain, A. (2008) Depression and diabetes in a rural community in Pakistan. *Diabetes Res. Clin. Pract.*, **79**, 124–127.

38. Chesla, C.A., Chun, K.M., and Kwan, C. (2009) Cultural and family challenges to managing type 2 diabetes in immigrant Chinese Americans. *Diabetes Care*, **32**, 1812–1816.

39. Fang, W., Weidong, W., Rongrui, Z. *et al.* (2008) Clinical observation on physiological and psychological effects of eight-section brocade on type 2 patient with diabetes. *J. Tradit. Chin. Med.*, **28**, 101–105.

40. Covington, M.B. (2001) Traditional Chinese medicine in the treatment of diabetes. *Diabetes Spectrum*, **14**, 154–159.

41. Flaskerud, J.H. and Calvillo, E.R. (2007) Cultural competence column psyche and soma: susto and diabetes. *Issues Ment. Health Nurs.*, **28**, 821–823.

42. Weller, S.C., Baer, R.D., Pachter, L.M. *et al.* (1999) Latino beliefs about diabetes. *Diabetes Care*, **22**, 722–728.

43. Fisher, L., Chesla, C.A., Mullan, J.T. *et al.* (2001) Contributors to depression in Latino and European-American patients with type 2 diabetes. *Diabetes Care*, **24**, 1751–1757.

44. Hsu, W.C., Cheung, S., Ong, E. *et al.* (2006) Identification of linguistic barriers to diabetes knowledge and glycemic control in Chinese Americans with diabetes. *Diabetes Care*, **29**, 415–416.

45. Ku, L. and Flores, G. (2005) Pay now or pay later: providing interpreter services in health care. *Health Aff.*, **24**, 435–444.

46. Leung, V.P.Y., Law, L.C.W., Chiu, H.F.K. *et al.* (2001) Validation study of the Chinese version of the Neuropsychiatric Inventory (CNPI). *Int. J. Geriatr. Psychiatry*, **16**, 789–793.

47. Yang, L.H. and Link, B.G. (1009) Comparing diagnostic methods for mental disorders in China. *Lancet*, **373**, 2002–2004.

48. Li, T.C., Lin, C.C., Liu, C.S., and Lee, Y.D. (2006) Validation of the Chinese version of the diabetes impact measurement scales amongst people suffering from diabetes. *Qual. Life Res.*, **15**, 1613–1619.

49. Shiu, A.T.Y., Wong, R.Y.M., and Thompson, D.R. (2003) Development of a reliable and valid Chinese version of the Diabetes Empowerment Scale. *Diabetes Care*, **26**, 2817–2821.

50. Huang, F.Y., Chung, H., Kroenke, K. *et al.* (2006) Using the Patient Health Questionnaire-9 to measure depression among racially and ethnically diverse primary care patients. *J. Gen. Intern. Med.*, **21**, 547–552.

51. Snoek, F.J. (2006) Diabetes and psychological well-being: crossing borders to achieve optimum care. *Pract. Diab. Int.*, **23**, 1–2.

52. Lustman, P.J. and Clouse, R.E. (2005) Depression in patient with diabetes: the relationship between mood and glycemic control. *J. Diabetes Complications*, **19**, 113–112.

53. Lustman, P.J., Griffith, L.S., Clouse, R.E., and Cryer, P.E. (1986) Psychiatric illness in diabetes mellitus. Relationship to symptoms and glucose control. *J. Nerv. Ment. Dis.*, **174**, 736–742.

54. Elderkin-Thompson, V., Hellemann, G., Gupta, R.K., and Kumar, A. (2009) Biophysical correlates of cognition among depressed and non-depressed type 2 diabetes patients. *Diabetes Care*, **32**, 48–50.

55. Kodl, C.T. and Seaquist, E.R. (2008) Cognitive dysfunction and diabetes mellitus. *Endocr. Rev.*, **29**, 494–511.

56. Lyoo, I.K., Yoon, S.J., Musen, G. *et al.* (2009) Altered prefrontal glutamate-glutamine-γ-aminobutyric acid levels and relation to low cognitive performance and depressive symptoms in type 1 diabetes mellitus. *Arch. Gen. Psychiatry*, **66**, 878–887.

57. Kumar, A., Gupta, R., Thomas, A. *et al.* (2009) Focal subcortical biophysical abnormalities in patients diagnosed with type 2 diabetes and depression. *Arch. Gen. Psychiatry*, **66**, 324–330.

58. Sommerfield, A.J., Deary, I.J., and Frier, B.M. (2004) Acute hyperglycemia alters mood state and impairs cognitive performance in people with type 2 diabetes. *Diabetes Care*, **27**, 2335–2340.

59. Lustman, P.J., Anderson, R.J., Freedland, K.E. *et al.* (2000) Depression and poor glycemic control. *Diabetes Care*, **23**, 934–942.

60. Cox, D.J., Kovatchev, B.P., Gonder-Frederick, L.A. *et al.* (2005) Relationships between hyperglycemia and cognitive performance among adults with type 1 and type 2 diabetes. *Diabetes Care*, **28**, 71–77.

61. Ryan, C.M., Freed, M.I., Rood, J.A. *et al.* (2006) Improving metabolic control leads to better working memory in adults with type 2 diabetes. *Diabetes Care*, **29**, 345–351.

62. Cox, D.J., Kovatchev, B., Vandecar, K. *et al.* (2006) Hypoglycemia preceding fatal car collisions. *Diabetes Care*, **29**, 467–468.

63. Ismail, K., Winkley, K., Stahl, D. *et al.* (2007) A cohort study of people with diabetes and their first foot ulcer. *Diabetes Care*, **30**, 1473–1479.

64. Iverse, M.M., Tell, G.S., Riise, T. *et al.* (2009) A history of foot ulcer increases mortality among persons with diabetes. 10-year follow-up of the Nord-TrøHealth Study, Norway. *Diabetes Care*, **32**, 2193–2199.

65. Clouse, R.E., Lustman, P.J., Feedland, K.E. *et al.* (2003) Depression and coronary heart disease in women with diabetes. *Psychosom. Med.*, **65**, 376–383.

66. Eason, S., Petersen, N., Suarez, M. *et al.* (2005) Diabetes mellitus, smoking, and the risk for asymptomatic peripheral arterial disease: whom should we screen? *J. Am. Board Fam. Pract.*, **18**, 355–361.

67. Blumenthal, J.A., Lett, H.S., Babyak, M.A. *et al.* (2003) Depression as a risk factor for mortality after coronary artery bypass surgery. *Lancet*, **362**, 604–609.

68. Lichtman, J.H., Bigger, J.T., Blumenthal, J.A. *et al.* (2008) Depression and coronary heart disease: recommendations for screening, referral, and treatment. *Circulation*, **118**, 1768–1775.

69. Whang, W. and Davidson, K.W. (2009) Is it time to treat depression in patients with cardiovascular disease? *Circulation*, **120**, 99–100.

70. Frasure-Smith, N., Lespérance, F., Habra, M. *et al.* (2009) Elevated depression symptoms predict long-term cardiovascular mortality in patients with atrial fibrillation and heart failure. *Circulation*, **120**, 134–140.

71. Arnold, S.V., Spertus, J.A., Ciechanowski, P.S. *et al.* (2009) Psychosocial modulators of angina response to myocardial ischemia. *Circulation*, **120**, 126–133.

72. Koopmans, B., Pouwer, F., de Bie, R.A. *et al.* (2009) Associations between vascular co-morbidities and depression in insulin-naive diabetes patients: the DIAZOB Primary Care Diabetes study. *Diabetologia*, **52**, 2056–2063.

73. Chen, Y.S., Wu, S.C., Wang, S.Y., and Jaw, B.S. (2003) Depression in chronic haemodialysed patients. *Nephrology*, **8**, 121–126.

74. Vileikyte, L., Leventhal, H., Gonzalez, J.S. *et al.* (2005) Diabetic peripheral neuropathy and depressive symptoms. *Diabetes Care*, **26**, 2378–2383.

75. Brands, A.M.A., Biessels, G.J., de Haan, E.H.F. *et al.* (2005) The effects of type 1 diabetes on cognitive performance. *Diabetes Care*, **28**, 726–735.

76. Munsen, G., Jacobson, A.M., Ryan, C.M. *et al.* (2008) The impact of diabetes and its treatment on cognitive function among adolescents who participated in the DCCT. *Diabetes Care*, **31**, 1933–1938.

77. Jacobson, A.M., Musen, G., Ryan, C.M. *et al.* (2007) Long-term effect of diabetes and its treatment on cognitive function. *N. Engl. J. Med.*, **356**, 1842–1852.

78. Bruehl, H., Rueger, M., Dziobek, I. *et al.* (2007) Hypothalamic-pituitary-adrenal axis dysregulation and memory impairments in type 2 diabetes. *J. Clin. Endocrinol. Metab.*, **92**, 2439–2445.

79. de Galan, B.E., Zoungas, S., Chalmers, J. *et al.* (2009) Cognitive function and risks of cardiovascular disease and hypoglycaemia in patients with type 2 diabetes: the ADVANCE trial. *Diabetologia*, **52**, 2328–2336.

80. Katon, W., Lin, E.H.B., and Ciechanowski, P. (2010) Comorbid depression is associated with an increased risk of dementia diagnosis in patients with diabetes: a prospective cohort study. *J. Gen. Intern. Med.*, **25**, 423–429.

81. Gonder-Frederick, L.A., Zrebiec, J.F., Bauchowitz, A.U. *et al.* (2009) Cognitive function is disrupted by both hypo- and hyperglycemia in school-aged children with type 1 diabetes: a field study. *Diabetes Care*, **32**, 1001–1006.

82. Ludman, E.J., Katon, W., Russo, J. *et al.* (2004) Depression and diabetes symptom burden. *Gen. Hosp. Psychiatry*, **26**, 430–436.

83. Lin, E.H.B., Katon, W., Von Korff, M. *et al.* (2004) Relationship of depression and diabetes self-care, medication adherence, and preventive care. *Diabetes Care*, **27**, 2154–2160.

84. U.S. Preventative Services Task Force (2009) Screening for depression in adults: U.S. Preventative Services Task Force recommendation statement. *Ann. Intern. Med.*, **151**, 784–792.

85. Pignone, M., Gaynes, B.N., Rushton, J.L. *et al.* (2002) Screening for depression; systematic evidence review. Agency for Healthcare Research and Quality, Rockville.

86. Pignone, M.P., Gaynes, B.N., Rushton, J.L. *et al.* (2002) Screening for depression in adults, a summary of the evidence for the U.S. Preventative Services Task Force. *Ann. Intern. Med.*, **136**, 765–776.

87. O'Connor, EA., Whitlock, EP., Gaynes, BN., and Beil, TL. (2009) Screening for depression in adults and older adults in primary care: an updated systematic review. Agency for Healthcare Research and Quality, Rockville.

88. Ryan, C.M., Freed, M.I., Rood, J.A. *et al.* (2006) Improving metabolic control leads to better working memory in adults with type 2 diabetes. *Diabetes Care*, **29**, 345–351.

89. Cox, D., Cox, D.J., Ford, D. *et al.* (2009) Driving mishaps among individuals with type 1 diabetes: a prospective study. *Diabetes Care*, **32**, 2177–2180.

90. O'Connor, E.A., Whitlock, E.P., Beil, T.L., and Gaynes, B.N. (2009) Screening for depression in adult patients in primary care settings: a systematic evidence review. *Ann. Intern. Med.*, **151**, 793–803.

91. Boyer, E.W. and Shannon, M. (2005) The serotonin syndrome. *N. Engl. J. Med.*, **352**, 1112–1120.

92. Rush, A.J., Trivedi, M.H., Wisniewski, S.R. *et al.* (2006) Acute and longer-term outcomes in depressed outpatients requiring one or several treatment steps: a STAR*D report. *Am. J. Psychiatry*, **163**, 1905–1927.

93. Williams, J.W., Jr., Mulrow, C.D., Chiquette, E. *et al.* (2000) A systematic review of newer pharmacotherapies for depression in adults: evidence report summary. *Ann. Intern. Med.*, **132**, 743–756.

94. Gurley, B., Swain, A., Williams, D.K. *et al.* (2008) Gauging the clinical significance of P-glycoprotein-mediated herb-drug interactions: comparative effects of St. John's wort, Echinacea, clarithromycin, and rifampin on digoxin pharmacokinetics. *Mol. Nutr. Food Res.*, **52**, 772–779.

95. de Abajo, F.J., Rodriguez, L.A., and Montero, D. (1999) Association between selective serotonin reuptake inhibitors and upper gastrointes-

tinal bleeding: population based case-control study. *BMJ*, **319**, 1106–1109.

96. van Walraven, C., Mamdani, M.M., Wells, P.S., and Williams, J.I. (2001) Inhibition of serotonin reuptake by antidepressants and upper gastrointestinal bleeding in elderly patients: retrospective cohort study. *BMJ*, **323**, 655–658.

97. Dalton, S.O., Johansen, C., Mellemkjaer, L. *et al.* (2003) Use of selective serotonin reuptake inhibitors and risk of upper gastrointestinal tract bleeding: a population-based cohort study. *Arch. Intern. Med.*, **163**, 59–64.

98. Richards, J.B., Papaioannou, A., Adachi, J.D. *et al.* (2007) Effect of selective serotonin reuptake inhibitors on the risk of fracture. *Arch. Intern. Med.*, **167**, 188–194.

99. Lustman, P.S., Clouse, R.E., and Carney, R.M. (1988) Depression and the reporting of diabetes symptoms. *Int. J. Psychiatry Med.*, **18**, 295–303.

100. Ciechanowski, P., Katon, W., Russo, J., and Hirsch, I. (2003) The relationship of depressive symptoms to symptom reporting, self-care and glucose control in diabetes. *Gen. Hosp. Psychiatry*, **25**, 246–252.

101. Spitzer, R., Kroenke, K., and Williams, J. (1999) Validation and utility of a self-report version of PRIME-MD: the PHQ primary care study. Primary care evaluation of mental disorders. Patient Health Questionnaire. *JAMA*, **282**, 1737–1744.

102. Polonsky, W.H., Fisher, L., Earles, J. *et al.* (2005) Assessing psychosocial stress in diabetes. *Diabetes Care*, **28**, 626–631.

103. Anderson, R.M. (1985) Is the problem of compliance all in our heads? *Diabetes Educ.*, **11**, 31–34.

104. Kilbourne, A.M., Reynold, C.F., Good, B. *et al.* (2005) How does depression influence diabetes medication adherence in older patients? *Am. J. Geriatr. Psychiatry*, **13**, 202–210.

105. Chao, J., Nau, D.P., Aikens, J.E., and Taylor, S.D. (2005) The mediating role of health beliefs in the relationship between depressive symptoms and medication adherence in persons with diabetes. *Res. Social Adm. Pharm.*, **1**, 508–525.

106. Colton, P.A., Olmsted, M.P., Daneman, D. *et al.* (2004) Disturbed eating behavior and eating disorders in preteen and early teenage girls with type 1 diabetes: a case controlled study. *Diabetes Care*, **27**, 1654–1659.

107. Crow, S., Kendall, D., Praus, B., and Thuras, P. (2000) Binge eating and other psychopathology in patients with type II diabetes mellitus. *Int. J. Eat. Disord.*, **30**, 222–226.

108. Jones, J.M., Lawson, M.L., Daneman, D. *et al.* (2000) Eating disorders in adolescent females with and without type 1 diabetes: cross sectional study. *BMJ*, **320**, 1563–1566.

109. Peveler, R.C., Bryden, K.S., Neil, H.A.W. *et al.* (2005) The relationship of disordered eating habits and attitudes to clinical outcomes in young adult females with type 1 diabetes. *Diabetes Care*, **28**, 84–88.

110. Morse, S., Ciechanowski, P.S., Katon, W.J., and Hirsch, I. (2006) Isn't this just bedtime snacking? The potential adverse effects of night eating symptoms on treatment adherence and outcomes in patients with diabetes. *Diabetes Care*, **29**, 1800–1804.

111. Pomerleau, C.S., Aubin, H.J., and Pomerleau, O.F. (1997) Self-reported alcohol use patterns in a sample of male and female heavy smokers. *J. Addict. Dis.*, **16**, 19–24.

112. Hall, S.M., Muñoz, R.F., Reus, V.I., and Sees, K.L. (1993) Nicotine, negative affect, and depression. *J. Consult. Clin. Psychol.*, **61**, 761–767.

113. Haire-Joshu, D., Heady, S., Thomas, L. *et al.* (1994) Depressive symptomatology and smoking among persons with diabetes. *Res. Nurs. Health*, **17**, 273–282.

114. Ciechanowski, P., Katon, W.J., and Russo, J.E. (2000) Depression and diabetes: impact of depressive symptoms on adherence, function and costs. *Arch. Intern. Med.*, **160**, 3278–3285.

115. Egede, L.E., Zheng, D., and Simpson, K. (2002) Comorbid depression is associated with increased health care use and expenditures in individuals with diabetes. *Diabetes Care*, **25**, 464–470.

116. Ciechanowski, P., Katon, W., Russo, J. *et al.* (2006) Where is the patient? The association of psychosocial factors with missed primary care appointments in patients with diabetes. *Gen. Hosp. Psychiatry*, **28**, 9–17.

117. Jacobson, A.M., Adler, A.G., Derby, L. *et al.* (1992) Clinic attendance and glycemic control. Study of contrasting groups of patients with IDDM. *Diabetes Care*, **14**, 599–601.

118. Karter, A.J., Parker, M.M., Moffet, H.H. *et al.* (2004) Missed appointments and poor glycemic control: an opportunity to identify high-risk diabetic patients. *Med. Care*, **42**, 110–115.

119. Hammersley, M.S., Holland, M.R., Walford, S., and Thorn, P.A. (1985) What happens to defaulters from a diabetic clinic? *BMJ*, **292**, 1330–1332.

120. Corsi, A., De-Castro, A., Ghisoni, G. *et al.* (1994) Reasons for patient dropout in attendance at diabetes clinics and evaluation of quality of care. *G. Ital. Diabetol.*, **14**, 239–242.

121. Griffin, S.J., (1998) Lost to follow-up: the problem of defaulters from diabetes clinics. *Diabet. Med.*, **15** (Suppl. 3), S14–S24.
122. Ciechanowski, P., Katon, W., and Russo, J. (2005) The association of depression and perceptions of interpersonal relationships in patients with diabetes. *J. Psychosom. Med.*, **58**, 139–144.
123. Ciechanowski, P., Russo, J., Katon, W. *et al.* (2004) Influence of patient attachment style on self-care and outcomes in diabetes. *Psychosom. Med.*, **66**, 720–728.
124. Mollema, E.D., Snoek, F.J., Adèr, H.J. *et al.* (2001) Insulin-treated diabetes patients with fear of self-injecting or fear of self-testing: psychological comorbidity and general well-being. *J. Psychosom. Res.*, **51**, 665–672.
125. Ciechanowski, P.S., Katon, W.J., Russo, J.E., and Walker, E.A. (2001) The patient-provider relationship: attachment theory and adherence to treatment in diabetes. *Am. J. Psychiatry*, **158**, 29–35.
126. Katon, W. and Unützer, J. (2006) Collaborative care models for depression: time to move from evidence to practice. *Arch. Intern. Med.*, **166**, 2304–2306.
127. Williams, J.W. Jr., Katon, W., Lin, E.H.B. *et al.* (2004) The effectiveness of depression care management on diabetes-related outcomes in older patients. *Ann. Intern. Med.*, **140**, 1015–1024.

# CHAPTER 6

# Depression and Diabetes: Sociodemographic and Cultural Aspects and Public Health Implications

**Juliana Chan**

*Hong Kong Institute of Diabetes and Obesity, Chinese University of Hong Kong, Prince of Wales Hospital, Hong Kong SAR, China Department of Medicine and Therapeutics, Chinese University of Hong Kong, Prince of Wales Hospital, Hong Kong SAR, China*

**Hairong Nan**

*Hong Kong Institute of Diabetes and Obesity, Chinese University of Hong Kong, Prince of Wales Hospital, Hong Kong SAR, China*

**Rose Ting**

*Department of Medicine and Therapeutics, Chinese University of Hong Kong, Prince of Wales Hospital, Hong Kong SAR, China*

The term 'culture' refers to the shared patterns of life that define social groups. Cultures are constantly subject to change. Social conflicts and development of technologies can produce societal changes by altering social dynamics and promoting new cultural models. Cultural ideas may transfer from one society to another through the process of acculturation, whereby immigrants adopt the attitudes, values, customs, beliefs and behaviours of a new culture.

*Depression and Diabetes* Edited by Wayne Katon, Mario Maj and Norman Sartorius
© 2010 John Wiley & Sons, Ltd

Even in the same ethnic group, people of different age, gender or living district may have different cultures. Cultural factors may affect the presentation, epidemiology, treatment modalities and outcomes of diseases, including diabetes and depression.

In 1985, only 30 million people worldwide were estimated to have diabetes. In 2000, the figure rose to over 150 million. In 2007, an estimated 7.3% of adults aged 20–79 years in International Diabetes Federation (IDF) member countries had diabetes. By 2025, the figure is expected to rise to 380 million [1]. Approximately 85–95% of affected people have type 2 diabetes in developed countries, and this type of diabetes possibly accounts for an even higher percentage in developing countries.

With increasing urbanization, millions of people are now living in urban or periurban areas. The effects of urbanization on health are mediated by increasing commercialism, acculturation and rapidly changing lifestyles. These include consumption of high calorie, high fat, high salt and low fibre diets, changing infant feeding practices, decreased physical activity, overcrowding and environmental contamination [2].

The diabetes epidemic is most rampant in non-European populations, as indicated by studies from Native American and Canadian communities, Pacific and Indian Ocean island populations, groups in India and Australian aboriginal communities [3].

The socioeconomic success of China has brought phenomenal lifestyle changes, with diabetes becoming a major public health problem [4]. In China, the prevalence of diabetes has increased from 1% in the early 1980s to 4.5% in the mid-1990s and 5.5% in the late 1990s [5–7], with higher rates in big cities like Beijing, Shanghai and Guangzhou than the rest of the country [8–11]. In a national survey conducted in 2007–2008, the prevalence of diabetes in China was estimated to be 10%, with middle-aged men as well as subjects with low education and socioeconomic status and obesity as major risk groups. Importantly, the most rapid increase in disease prevalence was observed in the young to middle-aged group, which will lead to an increasingly young population with or at risk of disabilities and premature mortality (Yang W.Y., personal communication).

Similarly, the scenario in India is changing rapidly, due to socio-economic transition in the rural areas. Better economic conditions have led to dramatic changes in dietary habits and declining physical activities, which have unmasked diabetes in a population likely to harbour genetic susceptibility, as evidenced by a lower threshold for risk factors including age, body mass index and upper body adiposity. In 2005, 33 million of people in India had diabetes, half of whom came from urban areas [12]. According to data from the IDF, the prevalence of diabetes in India will increase from 6.2% in 2007 to 7.6% in 2025 [13]. Recent epidemiological data suggest a narrowing urban–rural gradient in disease prevalence, with rising rates of metabolic syndrome and pre-diabetes, putting this population at high risk for diabetes and its complications [12].

Depression is an independent risk factor for the onset of type 2 diabetes. On the other hand, future risk for depression is also increased in patients with diabetes [14]. Depressive symptoms affect approximately one-quarter of the diabetic populations and are associated with suboptimal metabolic control, poor medication and diet adherence, reduced quality of life and increased healthcare expenditures [14, 15]. Among individuals with type 2 diabetes, minor and major depression is strongly associated with increased mortality [16]. In type 1 or 2 diabetic patients, the occurrence of depression is associated with increased risk of diabetic retinopathy, nephropathy, neuropathy, macrovascular complications and sexual dysfunction [17]. In the Hispanic Established Population for the Epidemiologic Study of the Elderly, diabetic patients with high level of depressive symptoms had 3.84 increased odds of death compared to those without depressive symptoms [18]. The longitudinal data from the same cohort showed the additive effects of diabetes and depression on increasing risk of premature mortality, earlier onset of macro/microvascular complications and disabilities in activities of daily living. These risk associations remained significant after controlling for sociodemographic characteristics including sex, age, education, acculturation and marital status [19].

## WOMEN, DEPRESSION AND DIABETES

Women with or without diabetes, irrespective of races, are at high risk for developing depression. They are three times more likely than men to have depression in response to any stressful events [20]. In a meta-analysis, Anderson *et al.* [21] reported the prevalence of depression in women with diabetes to be 27% compared to 18% in men. This gender difference is also evident in adolescence [22]. Keita summarized the risk factors for depression in women. Compared with men, women experience more negative life events, such as physical and sexual abuse, poverty, discrimination, and are more likely to have dependency on others [23]. Women also go through unique life stages, such as pregnancy and menopause, when hormonal and environmental factors may interact to trigger depression. Women of childbearing age are at heightened risk of experiencing a depressive episode. Approximately 10–20% of women experience depression during the postpartum period [24].

The relationships between gestational diabetes, maternal psychological distress and peripartum depression remain controversial. In a study which examined 100 pregnant women with diabetes or impaired glucose tolerance (IGT), although pregnant women with diabetes had a higher level of anxiety during their first assessment in the third trimester (around 30 weeks of gestation), this difference disappeared before the delivery and in the postpartum period [25].

In another study involving 11 024 pregnant women, among 657 women with pre-existing or gestational diabetes, 15.2% had depression during pregnancy or postpartum period. This was compared to 8.5% in women without diabetes. After adjusting for age, race, year of delivery and gestational age at birth, women with diabetes had nearly double the odds of experiencing depression during the perinatal period than their non-diabetic peers [26].

## DEPRESSION AND DIABETES IN LATE LIFE

With an aging population, the prevalence of diabetes is expected to rise, with increasing impact on the elderly health. Some investigators have argued that aging and rapid acculturation can lead to decline in growth hormone and sex steroids and activation of stress hormonal systems. These hormonal changes can lead to abnormal body composition, with increased deposition of visceral fat and cardio-metabolic risks [27]. Some authors have also reported an association of depressive symptoms with activation of the hypothalamic–pituitary–adrenal (HPA) axis [28] and increased inflammation [28–31]. Some patients with type 2 diabetes were reported to have increased serum cortisol and urinary catecholamine levels [32–34]. Apart from common pathways shared by diabetes and depression, suboptimal diabetes control can result in increased risk of micro/macrovascular complications, cognitive impairment, excessive skin problems and falls, the latter being also independently linked to depression and reduced quality of life in elderly [35].

There is a complex interplay between physical, cognitive, psychological and social factors in determining depression in the elderly. While physical disabilities, institutionalization, physical dependency and dementia are associated with high risk of depression in elderly, possibly due to cumulative life experiences and the development of healthier coping skills, adverse life events, neuroticism and social attachments are less important factors for depression in the elderly compared to the younger population.

Long-term intensive glycaemic control could lead to improvements in dementia, memory, energy, physical activity, mood and quality of life in the elderly. In light of the increasingly young age of onset of diabetes, early attainment of glycaemic control will have long-term benefits not only by reducing physical disabilities but also by preventing late-life depression. Thus, the importance of individualizing treatment goals, management strategies and appropriate use of pharmacotherapy cannot be overemphasized [35].

## SOCIOECONOMIC STATUS, DEPRESSION AND DIABETES

Low socioeconomic status is a common risk factor for depression and type 2 diabetes [36–38]. Depressed individuals are also more likely to smoke and gain weight, due to increased caloric intake and physical inactivity [39–41]. These psychological and behavioural factors interact to increase risk of diabetes and associated complications, particularly macrovascular ones [17]. The severity of these physical conditions in turn potentially adversely affects the psychological state, which influences physical well-being, thus setting up a vicious cycle.

The relationship between socioeconomic status, psychosocial factors and diabetes is complex. It is likely that socioeconomic status contributes to the development of diabetes through areas unrelated or indirectly related to psychosocial pathways, such as unhealthy lifestyles. The association between socioeconomic status and chronic diseases also tends to have opposite directions in developed and developing areas [38, 42, 43]. Thus, in low-resource areas, high personal affluence may lead to obesity and diabetes. By contrast, in developed countries, low socioeconomic status is often associated with inadequate health insurance, suboptimal preventive care, unhealthy lifestyle and poor access to healthcare, which collectively increase risk of diabetes and associated complications. Other social disadvantages and adverse life events can lead to high stress and give rise to symptoms such as depression, anxiety and hostility. The complex interplay among these risk factors may explain the frequent clustering of low socioeconomic status, poor physical and poor psychological health. Furthermore, the chronic stress of living in poverty and poor healthcare can set up a downward spiral with progressively deteriorating socioeconomic status resulting in unemployment, financial hardship and physical dependence.

In a population-based study with 23 years of follow-up [44], the risk of type 2 diabetes associated with major depressive disorder persisted over a life course, independent of health behaviours, body mass index and family history of diabetes, but education was found to be an important moderator of the risk association. Compared to subjects who never had major depressive disorder with high educational attainment, those who had major depressive disorder and low educational attainment had a 4.10-fold (95% CI = 1.84, 9.16) higher risk of diabetes, after adjusting for age, gender, race, smoking status, alcohol use, body mass index, family history of diabetes and social network.

Skodova *et al.* [45] identified 12 empirical studies which described socioeconomic determinants of cardiovascular risk factors and found that socioeconomic status – indicated by educational grade, occupation or income – was associated with an increased risk of cardiovascular disease. Low socioeconomic status was also associated with hostility and depression, lack of social support, poor perception of health and lack of optimism. More detailed studies are needed to explore the association of factors such as social network and family coherence on risk of diabetes and cardiovascular complications.

Given the importance of socioeconomic determinants in diabetes and cardiovascular disease, there is increasing advocacy to use an integrated approach to address psychological and socioeconomic health determinants in addition to conventional biomedical factors. The InterHeart Study [46] provided evidence in support of the universal pervasiveness of psychosocial and socioeconomic risk factors in determining cardiovascular disease. In this large survey, consisting of 24 767 participants from multiple ethnic groups in 52 countries, 33% of the population attributable risk of acute myocardial infarction was explained by variables pertinent to socioeconomic and lifestyle factors [46]. Despite this epidemiological evidence, the impact of addressing psychosocial factors or improving socioeconomic status on clinical outcome and quality of life remains unclear.

## MIGRATION, DIABETES AND DEPRESSION

The process of migration can be a triggering factor for depression. Studies have indicated a high prevalence of depression in migrants, due to multiple factors [47–49]. Migrants need to leave their original living place, which means loss of bonding and support with their family, friends and society. When they arrive in a new place, they face multiple stresses due to differences between their original and new cultures. Such stresses include culture shock (the stress reaction to an unfamiliar situation) and cultural conflicts. Migrants can be markedly distressed if they have an unrealistic expectation for achievement in a new environment. Finally, when migrants live long enough in the new environment, their own culture will gradually be assimilated by the major culture, so-called acculturation. When acculturation occurs on an involuntary base, this can give rise to strong emotional distress, resulting in social isolation and low self-esteem. On the other hand, migration can have a positive psychological impact on migrants, especially among those who appreciate the positive aspects of the majority culture [50].

Migration is associated with increased prevalence of diabetes in different ethnic groups during urbanization and modernization.

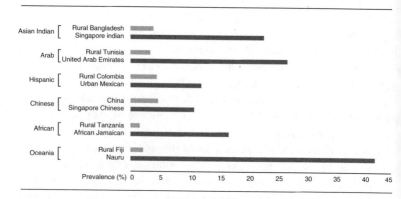

**Figure 6.1** Prevalence of type 2 diabetes among selected ethnic groups in 2007 (estimated by the International Diabetes Federation [13]).

Figure 6.1 shows the 10–40-fold higher prevalence of diabetes in migrants compared to their non-migrant peers within the same ethnic group living in different regions. Three major factors may contribute to this phenomenon. Urbanization associated with migration leads to major changes in dietary patterns, often characterized by high intake of energy dense foods, saturated fat and simple sugars and low intake of dietary fibres, fruits and vegetables. Physical inactivity usually occurs after modernization, with less engagement in labour-intensive jobs and an increasing switch to a sedentary lifestyle. Both nutritional transition and physical inactivity put people at high risk for obesity, metabolic syndrome and diabetes. Finally, migrants face multiple stresses which can lead to maladaptive responses, such as excessive smoking and alcoholic consumption, which trigger diabetes in later life [51].

## IMPACT OF ETHNICITY-RELATED CULTURE

### African Ancestry Groups

The African ancestry groups have a higher prevalence and a greater severity of diabetic complications than their white counterparts of the same age. In a meta-analysis, haemoglobin A1c (HbA1c) in Africans

Americans was higher than non-Hispanic whites by 0.65% [52]. Given that every 1% reduction in HbA1c is associated with a 21% risk reduction for any diabetes-related end point [53], a 0.65% HbA1c difference is clinically significant. In keeping with this finding, African Americans have a higher prevalence of diabetic retinopathy and are more likely to develop chronic kidney disease and end-stage renal failure requiring dialysis compared to their white counterparts [54–57].

The reasons for these inter-ethnic disparities in diabetes control and outcomes are multifactorial. The African Americans in general have worse health perception than whites. Chin *et al.* found that African American elderly often reported having a health problem for which they should have seen a doctor but did not [58]. Additionally, they reported lower rates of health insurance than the whites, with poor access to health care [52] resulting in delayed diagnoses and treatments. Compared to their white counterparts, African Americans are less likely to have HbA1c measurements, screening for diabetic retinopathy [58, 59] and prescription drug coverage [60].

Lack of social support, presence of medical illness and low levels of education are the most important predictors of high depressive symptoms in African Americans [61]. Other stressors, such as racist attitudes and discriminatory behaviour toward Africans, also make these ethnic groups vulnerable to mental disorders [62]. Misconceptions about causes of depression hinder early recognition and treatment of depression in this ethnic group. Many African Americans consider depression as a personal weakness rather than a health problem, with strong denial and perceived stigma. These attitudes often result in distrust of physicians, fewer uses of mental services and lower adherence to antidepressant medications [63–68] (Table 6.1).

## Asian Populations

The diabetes epidemic in Asia is considered to be a result of a complex interplay between genetic and environmental factors. For the same body mass index, Asians have a higher body fat percentage than

**Table 6.1** Characteristics of diabetes and depression in Africans, Asians and Latinos

|  | African | Asian | Latinos |
|---|---|---|---|
| *Diabetes* | High prevalence<br>More diabetic complications than white<br>Infrequent disease monitoring by patient or care professionals<br>Poor access to healthcare | Low body mass index despite high disease prevalence<br>Abdominal obesity is not uncommon<br>Rapid change from traditional to Westernized diet | High prevalence<br>More diabetic complications than white<br>Belief in *susto*<br>Rely on herbal remedies<br>Poor access to healthcare |
| *Depression* | Lack of social support<br>Low education level<br>Racism<br>Stigmatization<br>Misconceptions about depression | Masked by frequent somatization<br>Stigmatization<br>Family support<br>Determination to withstand hardship | Low socioeconomic status<br>Racism<br>Poor coping with acculturation<br>Low rates of receiving treatment<br>Family support |

non-Asians. Abdominal obesity (increased waist circumference and waist-to-hip ratio) is prevalent, especially in Southern Asians, which contributes to insulin resistance [69, 70]. These differences in body composition and insulin resistance interact with reduced early-phase insulin secretory capacity, resulting in glucose intolerance [71]. In the past two decades, Asia has undergone phenomenal economic development and urbanization. Rapid nutritional transition from a traditional diet to a 'Westernized diet' with high calorie, high animal fat and low fibre content [70, 72–75] is considered a major culprit for the rising epidemic of childhood obesity and increasingly early age of onset of diabetes in Asia.

This rising diabetes prevalence points to a looming epidemic of diabetic complications, including depression. There are major cultural differences between Asians and non-Asians in health beliefs regarding depression, adaptation to stresses and expression of psychological symptoms. Many Asian countries (especially the Far East Asian countries) share similar cultural backgrounds with China for historical reasons. Thus, understanding the cultural perspective of depression in the Chinese provides some insights into that of other Asian populations.

Several epidemiological studies have reported a lower rate of depression in Chinese than their Caucasian counterparts [76–80]. However, this is likely to be an underestimation, since the Chinese tend to express psychological distress with physical symptoms, such as headache, abdominal pain and fatigue. Many verbal expressions of the Chinese language do not discriminate between physical complaints and emotional distress. Hence, depressed individuals often report somatic symptoms to their doctors [81–85]. Besides, since emotional illness is not regarded as a disease by many Chinese, depressed individuals are less likely to seek medical advice or psychiatric services. Last but not least, Chinese culture perceives depression as a weakness of character and a cause of family shame, reducing the likelihood of it being detected early. In light of these cultural factors, Parker *et al.* [81] suggested interviewers to move from open-ended questions to specific questioning in order to detect depressive symptoms in the Chinese.

Stigmatization of depression is particularly strong in Chinese people, including those living outside China. Hsu *et al.* [86] assessed 50 foreign-born Chinese Americans' perception of stigmatization by asking them to read five case vignettes, covering diabetes, major depressive disorder, somatoform depression, psychotic depression and fever of unknown origin. They were asked to respond to 25 statements that contained six stigma factors. Compared with 50 Caucasian Americans, the stigma factor scores of both physical and mental illness were significantly higher among Chinese Americans, regardless of age, gender or educational level. Among the mental disorders, somatoform depression was less stigmatizing than major depressive disorder and psychotic depression in the Chinese American group.

Nonetheless, Chinese sociocultural factors may provide good protection against depression in patients with diabetes. Many Chinese were brought up to accept the need to withstand hardship and tolerate distressing circumstances with determination [81]. Much influenced by Confucianism, Chinese people have strong values for family well-being and stability, and often avoid open conflict to maintain family cohesion and harmony. In this connection, chronic disease management (including that of diabetes and depression) has been found to be more effective in families with good organization, low conflicts, high cohesion and stability of membership [87–89] (Table 6.1).

## Hispanic Populations

The Hispanics or Latinos are people of Cuban, Mexican, Puerto Rican, Dominican, South or Central American or other Spanish culture of origin regardless of race. They form a heterogeneous group but share similar core cultural beliefs and values. The Hispanics have become the second largest ethnic group in the United States, comprising 13.7% of the population. By the year 2050, Hispanics will represent around 25% of the United States population [90].

The prevalence of diabetes in Hispanic Americans is about 9.8%, while that in Caucasian Americans is 5.5%. As in other populations undergoing rapid transitions, a complex interplay between genetic and environmental factors is likely to contribute to the high prevalence of obesity and diabetes with an early age of onset in Hispanic Americans [91, 92]. Apart from sedentary lifestyle, excessive intake of calories and fat [93, 94], low socioeconomic status and education attainment are other risk factors for diabetes in Hispanic Americans [95].

Compared to their Caucasian counterparts, Hispanic Americans have higher rates of diabetic complications [96], including retinopathy, renal insufficiency and peripheral neuropathy [54, 57, 97, 98]. This is probably related to suboptimal glycaemic control [99], low education level and poor access to quality medical care. Other studies have shown that Hispanic Americans were less likely to attend doctors' visits or self-management classes or undergo dilated eye examinations [100, 101]. Many Hispanic Americans seldom or never performed self-monitoring of blood glucose [95], and their fondness for traditional high calorie, high fat Hispanic foods may be another barrier to their adherence to a healthy diet [102].

Hispanic adults believe that 'susto' increases one's susceptibility to diabetes. Susto means 'fright of surprise', which occurs during a specific startling event. The emotion can be fear, sadness, depression or joy [103, 104]. Once they develop diabetes, Hispanic Americans are more likely to report fatigue and mood changes than their Caucasian counterparts. Similar to Chinese, Hispanics emphasize family support during treatment, although some Hispanic subgroups believe weight reduction is not important or even harmful. They often prefer herbal remedies and hold negative attitudes toward insulin therapy, which they believe to signal onset of diabetes-related complications [105].

The prevalence of depression in the non-diabetic and diabetic Hispanics is similar to the Caucasian populations [106]. Precipitating factors for depression include low socioeconomic status, racism; financial, occupational and social hardships; difficulty to adapt during acculturation and discrimination. Nevertheless, their strong family relationships and ease in interpersonal relationships, to some extent, protect them from depression [106, 107].

Similar to African Americans, Hispanics have lower rates of treatment for depression, regardless of their insurance and socio-demographic status [68, 108, 109]. They have insufficient knowledge and different attitudes about depression and are less likely to seek active treatment. Therefore, culturally sensitive education strategies are needed to empower patients and their family to learn about these diseases, in order to change their attitudes and social norms so as to improve their moods and behaviours (Table 6.1).

## MEASURES TO REDUCE HEALTH DISPARITIES AMONG PEOPLE FROM DIFFERENT CULTURAL BACKGROUNDS

Communities such as those with low socioeconomic status, including minority ethnic groups, suffer from a disproportionate burden of diabetes and depression. Hence, effective treatment and intervention targeted at these high risk groups are crucial to reduce racial disparities in health outcomes. However, such intervention strategies need to take into consideration the diverse cultural backgrounds of these communities. While multilevel measures targeted at patients, care providers and health systems are often advocated to reduce disparities of health outcomes, there remains a scarcity of data on the implementation and cost effectiveness of such interventions.

There is some evidence supporting the use of interventions that target patients (primarily through culturally tailored programmes), providers (especially through one-on-one feedback and education), health systems (particularly with nurse case managers and nurse clinicians, or telephone follow-up counselling) [110–113]. The use of peer support to motivate behavioural changes and manage negative emotions in people with chronic diseases such as diabetes and depression is gaining international attention. Given the worldwide nature of these epidemics, it remains a huge challenge to launch these global peer support programmes. Nevertheless, creating a global network of peer support may shed light on its contributions to health in different cultures and environments. Such a network also has the potential to enhance diabetes awareness within the community and among care professionals on how peer support is shaped by its contexts in cultures, families, neighbourhoods and healthcare systems [114].

Healthcare providers are important determinants for quality of healthcare and outcomes. Training healthcare providers on the cultural needs of ethnic minorities reduces the barrier of clinical inertia (the lack of treatment intensification despite clinical indications) during treatment of such patients [110]. Interventions to providers are mainly carried out through education activities. These include cultural competency training, issuing practice guidelines, continuing medical education, computerized decision support reminders, problem-based learning and in-person feedback [115–117]. Among these interventions, in-person feedback to providers has been shown to be successful in sustaining provider behavioural changes and improving health outcomes in diabetes [115–117].

Interventions at the level of the healthcare system include the use of disease management and non-physician providers to deliver care. Some studies indicated that use of registered nurses to deliver care significantly improved clinical outcomes in people with diabetes [118–120]. A study evaluated the use of an automated, self-assisted telephone disease management system by patients followed by telephone calls by nurses as a strategy to improve outcomes including HbA1c, mental health, self-efficacy, satisfaction with care and health-related quality of life among low-income patients with diabetes in the United States [118, 119]. Researchers enrolled 280 English- or Spanish-speaking adults with diabetes who were using hypoglycaemic medications and were treated in a county healthcare system. Patients were randomly assigned to usual care (control group) or to receive an intervention that consisted of usual care plus biweekly automated assessment and self-care education calls with telephone follow-up by a nurse educator. Outcomes measured at 12 months included survey-reported self-care, perceived glycaemic control, symptoms and HbA1c levels. Compared with the control group, patients in the intervention group reported fewer symptoms of depression (p = 0.023), greater self-efficacy to conduct self-care activities (p = 0.006) and fewer days in bed because of illness (p = 0.026) at follow-up. In these patients, HbA1c level was 0.3% lower than control group, albeit short of significance.

Other studies have also demonstrated the benefits of pharmacist-led medication management and patient education programmes on increasing diabetes knowledge with enhanced patient satisfaction [112, 121]. Despite these positive results, there is a need to link or integrate these intervention programmes to clinical care to avoid gaps and overlaps. Furthermore, interventions by care professionals can be labour intensive and costly, which may limit their generalized use in real practice, especially in low resource areas. Here, use of trained community health workers and peer supporters may be an alternative to overcome the social, cultural and linguistic barriers in different ethnic groups [110].

Nowadays, the news media and Internet are important sources of information on health and health policy. They can shape the public's opinions about issues by emphasizing certain features in their coverage, such as the causes of a problem, who is responsible for addressing it and what groups are affected. Gollust and Lantz [122] analysed data from 698 print news articles in 19 US newspapers between 2005 and 2006 and found that the predominant explanation for type 2 diabetes was behavioural factors and obesity. Less than 12% of the articles described social determinants, upstream policy solutions and disparities in diabetes. The disproportionately greater burden of chronic diseases in ethnic minorities and socioeconomically disadvantaged groups was rarely mentioned. These findings suggest the potential to use mass media to increase public awareness of disparities and social determinants of chronic diseases, as well as to engage the public to support policies to improve population health.

In some developed countries, media initiatives including the Internet and educational programmes, such as the National Screening Day for Depression and World Diabetes Day, are used to promote public awareness and positive attitudes towards these chronic diseases [123].

In addition to health promotion, early detection programmes are frequently advocated, especially if there are valid screening tests. Given their frequent coexistence, healthcare professionals are encouraged to screen for depression in people with diabetes or diabetes/prediabetes in people with depressive disorders [81–83, 124]. In the treatment of chronic diseases, multidisciplinary teams and patient registries are often used to implement and evaluate effectiveness of prevention strategies. These include patient education and case management by nurses, treatment algorithms, outreach programmes by community health workers, group visits, patient incentives and continuous quality improvement schemes [110, 125]. Both systematic reviews and meta-analyses have confirmed the benefits of using paramedics such as nurses and pharmacists to deliver care protocols in patients with chronic diseases such as diabetes, heart failure and cardio-renal complications. Components of these protocols often include telephone counselling, review by paramedics and periodic assessments to ensure the continuum of care [111–113].

Other public health experts propose the use of peer support to improve management of patients with chronic diseases such as diabetes and depression. Here, peers fulfil three important functions by providing assistance in managing and living with these chronic diseases on a daily basis, social and emotional support and linkage to clinical care. Guided by these principles, programmes can be further modified depending on resources, support, setting feasibility and patients' perspectives [114]. While there are reports showing the beneficial effects of peer support, there remain multiple challenges. These include promoting peer intervention as part of routine chronic care, linking them to the healthcare system and harmonizing the roles of peers with family, care professionals and other social networks in these prevention programmes [114]. Despite these uncertainties, in a recent randomized study, the use of peer support has been shown to reduce the incidence of postpartum depression among high risk women [126]. These studies highlight the values of using nurses and trained peers, who are often more appreciative of the individual needs of patients with diabetes and depression.

Cost-containing measures imposed by health maintenance organizations have limited the availability of early detection programmes and access of patients to specialty care and better tolerated treatments. Facing the rising burden of chronic diseases at an increasingly young age of onset, policy makers have major challenges to contain healthcare expenditures without compromising the quality of care.

Many unhealthy habits are deeply rooted and highly prevalent, especially in developing areas, in part due to poor education and unfavourable living environment. Unhealthy lifestyles do not exist in isolation, but are closely related to social and physical circumstances in which people are born, raised and spend their lives. Thus, it is unlikely that simple interventions can deal with health disparities with multiple determinants [125]. On the other hand, the use of a variety of tools through multisectoral efforts is more likely to change lifestyle, cultural norms, and living and working environments to promote and improve health.

For example, to control depression, there is a need to improve access to care, ensure proper evaluation, initiation and completion of treatment. Importantly, systems must be put in place to ensure appropriate payment for these treatments [125]. Some of the most powerful diabetes interventions targeted patients, providers, organizations and community factors simultaneously [110]. To facilitate the propagation of best practices which can be customized to suit local needs, a central system can be developed to collect, assess and disseminate information about health promotion and disease prevention. Furthermore, healthcare payers (e.g. health insurers) and providers must be given incentives to develop and support 'evidence-based' preventive activities both inside and outside the traditional care domain such as hospitals and clinics. Such a system can be augmented by ongoing interactions among researchers, policy makers, healthcare administrators, care professionals and affected individuals to complete the cycle of research, practice and policy to achieve better health outcomes.

## INTERVENTION STRATEGIES AND RESEARCH DIRECTIONS FOR TRANSCULTURAL HEALTH NEEDS

With increasing globalization and urbanization, healthcare providers will face increasing challenges to treat depression in people with different cultural backgrounds and social contexts. Thus, it is a public health priority to train physicians to recognize the heterogeneity of clinical presentations of depression in patients with different ethnic and cultural backgrounds. However, there are only a few studies which compare culturally tailored interventions to generic quality improvement programmes to address the specific needs of minority or ethnic groups with diabetes and depression. Here, barriers relating to individuals, communities and healthcare organizations need to be addressed. Despite the lack of evidence, there are theoretical and practical reasons to believe that such cultural tailoring may enhance the effectiveness of intervention in these subjects, with possible narrowing of the health inequality [125]. Herein, culturally tailored education materials and psychotherapy delivered by trained healthcare personnel, with or without peer support, may overcome the stigma of mental illnesses and stresses associated with discrimination, racism and acculturation. The use of ethnic-matched providers who are culturally and linguistically representative of the minority ethnic communities, provision of translation services and culturally sensitive patient information materials, use of outreach programmes and home visits are other measures used to address transcultural healthcare needs. The traditional training of nurses to work in teams with particular focus on patients' needs puts them in an ideal position to deliver culturally sensitive prevention and care programmes [125]. Against this background, evaluation of the cost effectiveness of prevention programmes in diabetes and/or depression is an emerging field. As such, there is a need to develop and validate the utility of prevention strategies tailored to meet the pluralistic needs of communities with diverse cultural backgrounds and different stages of socioeconomical development.

## CONCLUSIONS

The double burden of diabetes and depression, in part driven by rapid modernization and acculturation, is escalating healthcare expenditures, reducing societal productivity and causing personal and family suffering. These diseases are highly prevalent in non-white populations undergoing rapid acculturation and in indigenous or ethnic minority groups living in modern societies with major health inequalities. Factors pertinent to specific cultures (e.g. languages, beliefs and habits), socioeconomic factors (e.g. education levels, employment, living and working environments) and access to care are some of the factors which may contribute to these health disparities.

From a public health perspective, primary prevention strategies aim to reduce exposure of the whole population to risk factors through changing environments and health-promoting policies, such as anti-smoking and nutritional labelling campaigns. In secondary prevention, strategies are used to detect cases early for intervention. While there are theoretical reasons to believe that culturally sensitive care and control programmes for chronic diseases such as diabetes and depression should be effective, there is a paucity of data on the implementation and evaluation of such programmes. In light of the rising burden of chronic diseases affecting mainly non-white populations, such data are urgently needed to assess needs, strengthen capacity and eventually introduce policy to make these intervention programmes accessible, sustainable and affordable.

## REFERENCES

1. International Diabetes Federation. Diabetes prevalence. http://www.idf.org.
2. Gracey, M. (2002) Child health in an urbanizing world. *Acta Paediatr.*, **91**, 1–8.
3. Zimmet, P., Alberti, K.G., and Shaw, J. (2001) Global and societal implications of the diabetes epidemic. *Nature*, **414**, 782–787.

4. Wild, S., Roglic, G., Green, A. *et al.* (2004) Global prevalence of diabetes: estimates for the year 2000 and projections for 2030. *Diabetes Care*, **27**, 1047–1053.

5. National Diabetes Co-operative Study Group (1981) A mass survey of diabetes mellitus in a population of 300 000 in 14 provinces and municipalities in China. *Chinese J. Int. Med.*, **20**, 678–683.

6. Wang, K., Li, T., and Xiang, H.D. (1998) Study on the epidemiological characteristics of diabetes mellitus and IGT in China. *Zhonghua Liu Xing Bing Xue Za Zhi*, **19**, 282–285.

7. Gu, D., Reynolds, K., Duan, X. *et al.* (2003) Prevalence of diabetes and impaired fasting glucose in the Chinese adult population: International Collaborative Study of Cardiovascular Disease in Asia (InterASIA). *Diabetologia*, **46**, 1190–1198.

8. Beijing Diabetes Research Cooperative Group (1982) The prevalence of diabetes mellitus in 40,000 population in Beijing with discussion on different criteria for its diagnosis. *Zhonghua Nei Ke Za Zhi*, **21**, 85–87.

9. Diabetes Research Cooperation Group (2002) A survey of diabetes prevalence in middle aged and elderly Chinese from 12 areas of China. *Chin. J. Endocrinol. Metab.*, **18**, 280–284.

10. Jia, W.P., Xiang, K.S., Chen, L. *et al.* (2002) Epidemiological study on obesity and its comorbidities in urban Chinese older than 20 years of age in Shanghai, China. *Obes. Rev.*, **3**, 157–165.

11. Dong, Y., Gao, W., Nan, H. *et al.* (2005) Prevalence of type 2 diabetes in urban and rural Chinese populations in Qingdao, China. *Diabet. Med.*, **22**, 1427–1433.

12. Ramachandran, A. (2005) Epidemiology of diabetes in India – three decades of research. *J. Assoc. Physicians India*, **53**, 34–38.

13. International Diabetes Federation. Diabetes Atlas: South East Asian Region. http://www.idf.org.

14. Lustman, P.J. and Clouse, R.E. (2005) Depression in diabetic patients: the relationship between mood and glycemic control. *J. Diabetes Complications*, **19**, 113–122.

15. Goldney, R.D., Phillips, P.J., Fisher, L.J., and Wilson, D.H. (2004) Diabetes, depression, and quality of life: a population study. *Diabetes Care*, **27**, 1066–1070.

16. Katon, W.J., Rutter, C., Simon, G. *et al.* (2005) The association of comorbid depression with mortality in patients with type 2 diabetes. *Diabetes Care*, **28**, 2668–2672.

17. de Groot, M., Anderson, R., Freedland, K.E. *et al.* (2001) Association of depression and diabetes complications: a meta-analysis. *Psychosom. Med.*, **63**, 619–630.

18. Black, S.A. and Markides, K.S. (1999) Depressive symptoms and mortality in older Mexican Americans. *Ann. Epidemiol.*, **9**, 45–52.

19. Black, S.A., Markides, K.S., and Ray, L.A. (2003) Depression predicts increased incidence of adverse health outcomes in older Mexican Americans with type 2 diabetes. *Diabetes Care*, **26**, 2822–2828.

20. Maciejewski, P.K., Prigerson, H.G., and Mazure, C.M. (2001) Sex differences in event-related risk for major depression. *Psychol. Med.*, **31**, 593–604.

21. Anderson, R.J., Freedland, K.E., Clouse, R.E., and Lustman, P.J. (2001) The prevalence of comorbid depression in adults with diabetes: a meta-analysis. *Diabetes Care*, **24**, 1069–1078.

22. Kuehner, C. (2003) Gender differences in unipolar depression: an update of epidemiological findings and possible explanations. *Acta Psychiatr. Scand.*, **108**, 163–174.

23. Keita, G.P. (2007) Psychosocial and cultural contributions to depression in women: considerations for women midlife and beyond. *J. Manag. Care Pharm.*, **13**, S12–S15.

24. Clay, E.C. and Seehusen, D.A. (2004) A review of postpartum depression for the primary care physician. *South Med. J.*, **97**, 157–161.

25. Daniells, S., Grenyer, B.F., Davis, W.S. *et al.* (2003) Gestational diabetes mellitus: is a diagnosis associated with an increase in maternal anxiety and stress in the short and intermediate term? *Diabetes Care*, **26**, 385–389.

26. Kozhimannil, K.B., Pereira, M.A., and Harlow, B.L. (2009) Association between diabetes and perinatal depression among low-income mothers. *JAMA*, **301**, 842–847.

27. Bjorntorp, P. (1991) Metabolic implications of body fat distribution. *Diabetes Care*, **14**, 1132–1143.

28. Musselman, D.L., Betan, E., Larsen, H., and Phillips, L.S. (2003) Relationship of depression to diabetes types 1 and 2: epidemiology, biology, and treatment. *Biol. Psychiatry*, **54**, 317–329.

29. Black, P.H. (2003) The inflammatory response is an integral part of the stress response: implications for atherosclerosis, insulin resistance, type II diabetes and metabolic syndrome X. *Brain Behav. Immun.*, **17**, 350–364.

30. Ford, D.E. and Erlinger, T.P. (2004) Depression and C-reactive protein in US adults: data from the Third National Health and Nutrition Examination Survey. *Arch. Intern. Med.*, **164**, 1010–1014.

31. Kiecolt-Glaser, J.K. and Glaser, R. (2002) Depression and immune function: central pathways to morbidity and mortality. *J. Psychosom. Res.*, **53**, 873–876.

32. Lee, Z.S., Chan, J.C., Yeung, V.T. *et al.* (1999) Plasma insulin, growth hormone, cortisol, and central obesity among young Chinese type 2 diabetic patients. *Diabetes Care*, **22**, 1450–1457.

33. Kong, A.P., Chan, N.N., and Chan, J.C. (2006) The role of adipocytokines and neurohormonal dysregulation in metabolic syndrome. *Curr. Diabetes Rev.*, **2**, 397–407.

34. Lee, Z.S., Critchley, J.A., Tomlinson, B. *et al.* (2001) Urinary epinephrine and norepinephrine interrelations with obesity, insulin, and the metabolic syndrome in Hong Kong Chinese. *Metabolism*, **50**, 135–143.

35. Drab, S.R. (2009) Recognizing the rising impact of diabetes in seniors and implications for its management. *Consult Pharm.*, **24** (Suppl. B), 5–10.

36. Steptoe, A., Owen, N., Kunz-Ebrecht, S., and Mohamed-Ali, V. (2002) Inflammatory cytokines, socioeconomic status, and acute stress responsivity. *Brain Behav. Immun.*, **16**, 774–784.

37. Jousilahti, P., Salomaa, V., Rasi, V. *et al.* (2003) Association of markers of systemic inflammation, C reactive protein, serum amyloid A, and fibrinogen, with socioeconomic status. *J. Epidemiol. Community Health*, **57**, 730–733.

38. Ko, G.T., Chan, J.C., Yeung, V.T. *et al.* (2001) A low socio-economic status is an additional risk factor for glucose intolerance in high risk Hong Kong Chinese. *Eur. J. Epidemiol.*, **17**, 289–295.

39. Carnethon, M.R., Biggs, M.L., Barzilay, J.I. *et al.* (2007) Longitudinal association between depressive symptoms and incident type 2 diabetes mellitus in older adults: the Cardiovascular Health Study. *Arch. Intern. Med.*, **167**, 802–807.

40. Golden, S.H., Williams, J.E., Ford, D.E. *et al.* (2004) Depressive symptoms and the risk of type 2 diabetes: the Atherosclerosis Risk in Communities study. *Diabetes Care*, **27**, 429–435.

41. Engum, A. (2007) The role of depression and anxiety in onset of diabetes in a large population-based study. *J. Psychosom. Res.*, **62**, 31–38.

42. Xu, F., Yin, X.M., Zhang, M. *et al.* (2006) Family average income and diagnosed type 2 diabetes in urban and rural residents in regional mainland China. *Diabet. Med.*, **23**, 1239–1246.

43. Connolly, V., Unwin, N., Sherriff, P. *et al.* (2000) Diabetes prevalence and socioeconomic status: a population based study showing increased prevalence of type 2 diabetes mellitus in deprived areas. *J. Epidemiol. Community Health*, **54**, 173–177.

44. Mezuk, B., Eaton, W.W., Golden, S.H., and Ding, Y. (2008) The influence of educational attainment on depression and risk of type 2 diabetes. *Am. J. Public Health*, **98**, 1480–1485.

45. Skodova, Z., Nagyova, I., van Dijk, J.P. *et al.* (2008), Socioeconomic differences in psychosocial factors contributing to coronary heart disease: a review. *J. Clin. Psychol. Med. Settings,* **15,** 204–213.

46. Rosengren, A., Hawken, S., Ounpuu S., *et al.* (2004) Association of psychosocial risk factors with risk of acute myocardial infarction in 11 119 cases and 13 648 controls from 52 countries (the INTERHEART study): case-control study. *Lancet*, **364**, 953–962.

47. Graco, M., Berlowitz, D.J., Fourlanos, S., and Sundram, S. (2009) Depression is greater in non-English speaking hospital outpatients with type 2 diabetes. *Diabetes Res. Clin. Pract.*, **83**, e51–e53.

48. Oei, T.P. and Notowidjojo, F. (1990) Depression and loneliness in overseas students. *Int. J. Soc. Psychiatry*, **36**, 121–130.

49. Lai, D.W. (2004) Depression among elderly Chinese-Canadian immigrants from Mainland China. *Chin. Med. J.*, **117**, 677–683.

50. Bhugra, D. and Becker, M.A. (2005) Migration, cultural bereavement and cultural identity. *World Psychiatry*, **4**, 18–24.

51. Misra, A. and Ganda, O.P. (2007) Migration and its impact on adiposity and type 2 diabetes. *Nutrition*, **23**, 696–708.

52. Kirk, J.K., D'Agostino, R.B. Jr., Bell, R.A. *et al.* (2006) Disparities in HbA1c levels between African-American and non-Hispanic white adults with diabetes: a meta-analysis. *Diabetes Care*, **29**, 2130–2136.

53. Stratton, I.M., Adler, A.I., Neil, H.A. *et al.* (2000) Association of glycaemia with macrovascular and microvascular complications of type 2 diabetes (UKPDS 35): prospective observational study. *BMJ*, **321**, 405–412.

54. Harris, M.I., Klein, R., Cowie, C.C. *et al.* (1998) Is the risk of diabetic retinopathy greater in non-Hispanic blacks and Mexican Americans than in non-Hispanic whites with type 2 diabetes? A U.S. population study. *Diabetes Care*, **21**, 1230–1235.

55. Young, B.A., Maynard, C., and Boyko, E.J. (2003) Racial differences in diabetic nephropathy, cardiovascular disease, and mortality in a national population of veterans. *Diabetes Care*, **26**, 2392–2399.

56. Young, B.A., Pugh, J.A., Maynard, C., and Reiber, G. (2004) Diabetes and renal disease in veterans. *Diabetes Care*, **27** (Suppl. 2), B45–B49.

57. Carter, J.S., Pugh, J.A., and Monterrosa, A. (1996) Non-insulin-dependent diabetes mellitus in minorities in the United States. *Ann. Intern. Med.*, **125**, 221–232.

58. Chin, M.H., Zhang, J.X., and Merrell, K. (1998) Diabetes in the African-American Medicare population. Morbidity, quality of care, and resource utilization. *Diabetes Care*, **21**, 1090–1095.

59. Trivedi, A.N., Zaslavsky, A.M., Schneider, E.C., and Ayanian, J.Z. (2005) Trends in the quality of care and racial disparities in Medicare managed care. *N. Engl. J. Med.*, **353**, 692–700.

60. Briesacher, B., Limcangco, R., and Gaskin, D. (2003) Racial and ethnic disparities in prescription coverage and medication use. *Health Care Financ. Rev.*, **25**, 63–76.

61. Okwumabua, J.O., Baker, F.M., Wong, S.P., and Pilgram, B.O. (1997) Characteristics of depressive symptoms in elderly urban and rural African Americans. *J. Gerontol. A Biol. Sci. Med. Sci.*, **52**, M241–M246.

62. Gary, T.L., Crum, R.M., Cooper-Patrick, L. *et al.* (2000) Depressive symptoms and metabolic control in African-Americans with type 2 diabetes. *Diabetes Care*, **23**, 23–29.

63. Egede, L.E. (2002) Beliefs and attitudes of African Americans with type 2 diabetes toward depression. *Diabetes Educ.*, **28**, 258–268.

64. Wagner, J., Tsimikas, J., Abbott, G. *et al.* (2007) Racial and ethnic differences in diabetic patient-reported depression symptoms, diagnosis, and treatment. *Diabetes Res. Clin. Pract.*, **75**, 119–122.

65. Spencer, M.S., Kieffer, E.C., Sinco, B.R. *et al.* (2006) Diabetes-specific emotional distress among African Americans and Hispanics with type 2 diabetes. *J. Health Care Poor Underserved*, **17**, 88–105.

66. Padgett, D.K., Patrick, C., Burns, B.J., and Schlesinger, H.J. (1994) Ethnicity and the use of outpatient mental health services in a national insured population. *Am. J. Public Health*, **84**, 222–226.

67. de Groot, M. and Lustman, P.J. (2001) Depression among African-Americans with diabetes: a dearth of studies. *Diabetes Care*, **24**, 407–408.

68. Skaer, T.L., Sclar, D.A., Robison, L.M., and Galin, R.S. (2000) Trends in the rate of depressive illness and use of antidepressant pharmacotherapy by ethnicity/race: an assessment of office-based visits in the United States 1992–1997. *Clin. Ther.*, **22**, 1575–1589.

69. Park, Y.W., Allison, D.B., Heymsfield, S.B., and Gallagher, D. (2001) Larger amounts of visceral adipose tissue in Asian Americans. *Obes. Res.*, **9**, 381–387.

70. Chan, J.C., Malik, V., Jia, W. *et al.* (2009) Diabetes in Asia: epidemiology, risk factors, and pathophysiology. *JAMA*, **301**, 2129–2140.

71. Yoon, K.H., Lee, J.H., Kim, J.W. *et al.* (2006) Epidemic obesity and type 2 diabetes in Asia. *Lancet*, **368**, 1681–1688.

72. Seidell, J.C. (2000) Obesity, insulin resistance and diabetes – a worldwide epidemic. *Br. J. Nutr.*, **83** (Suppl. 1), S5–S8.

73. Popkin, B.M., Horton, S., Kim, S. *et al.* (2001) Trends in diet, nutritional status, and diet-related noncommunicable diseases in China and India: the economic costs of the nutrition transition. *Nutr. Rev.*, **59**, 379–390.

74. Popkin, B.M. and Du, S. (2003) Dynamics of the nutrition transition toward the animal foods sector in China and its implications: a worried perspective. *J. Nutr.*, **133**, 3898S–3906S.

75. Hosler, A.S. and Melnik, T.A. (2003) Prevalence of diagnosed diabetes and related risk factors: Japanese adults in Westchester County, New York. *Am. J. Public Health*, **93**, 1279–1281.

76. Kessler, R.C., Chiu, W.T., Demler, O. *et al.* (2005) Prevalence, severity, and comorbidity of 12-month DSM-IV disorders in the National Comorbidity Survey Replication. *Arch. Gen. Psychiatry*, **62**, 617–627.

77. Takeuchi, D.T., Chung, R.C., Lin, K.M. *et al.* (1998) Lifetime and twelve-month prevalence rates of major depressive episodes and dysthymia among Chinese Americans in Los Angeles. *Am. J. Psychiatry*, **155**, 1407–1414.

78. Golden, S.H., Lazo, M., Carnethon, M. *et al.* (2008) Examining a bidirectional association between depressive symptoms and diabetes. *JAMA*, **299**, 2751–2759.

79. Chen, C.N., Wong, J., Lee, N. *et al.* (1993) The Shatin community mental health survey in Hong Kong. II. Major findings. *Arch. Gen. Psychiatry*, **50**, 125–133.

80. Lee, S., Tsang, A., and Kwok, K. (2007) Twelve-month prevalence, correlates, and treatment preference of adults with DSM-IV major depressive episode in Hong Kong. *J. Affect. Disord.*, **98**, 129–136.

81. Parker, G., Gladstone, G., and Chee, K.T. (2001) Depression in the planet's largest ethnic group: the Chinese. *Am. J. Psychiatry*, **158**, 857–864.

82. Kleinman, A. (1982) Neurasthenia and depression: a study of somatization and culture in China. *Cult. Med. Psychiatry*, **6**, 117–190.

83. Kleinman, A. (2004) Culture and depression. *N. Engl. J. Med.*, **351**, 951–953.

84. Hsu, L.K. and Folstein, M.F. (1997) Somatoform disorders in Caucasian and Chinese Americans. *J. Nerv. Ment. Dis.*, **185**, 382–387.

85. Xu, J.M. (1987) Some issues in the diagnosis of depression in China. *Can. J. Psychiatry*, **32**, 368–370.

86. Hsu, L.K., Wan, Y.M., Chang, H. *et al.* (2008) Stigma of depression is more severe in Chinese Americans than Caucasian Americans. *Psychiatry*, **71**, 210–218.

87. Cox, D.J. and Gonder-Frederick, L. (1992) Major developments in behavioral diabetes research. *J. Consult. Clin. Psychol.*, **60**, 628–638.

88. Fisher, L., Chesla, C.A., Skaff, M.M. *et al.* (2000) The family and disease management in Hispanic and European-American patients with type 2 diabetes. *Diabetes Care*, **23**, 267–272.

89. Trief, P.M., Grant, W., Elbert, K., and Weinstock, R.S. (1998) Family environment, glycemic control, and the psychosocial adaptation of adults with diabetes. *Diabetes Care*, **21**, 241–245.

90. US Census Bureau. Annual estimates of the resident population by sex, race, and Hispanic origin for the United States: April 1, 2000 to July 1, 2008. www.census.gov.

91. Neel, J.V. (1962) Diabetes mellitus: a "thrifty" genotype rendered detrimental by "progress"? *Am. J. Hum. Genet.*, **14**, 353–362.

92. Ogden, C.L., Carroll, M.D., Curtin, L.R. *et al.* (2006) Prevalence of overweight and obesity in the United States, 1999–2004. *JAMA*, **295**, 1549–1555.

93. Wilbur, J., Chandler, P.J., Dancy, B., and Lee, H. (2003) Correlates of physical activity in urban Midwestern African-American women. *Am. J. Prev. Med.*, **25**, 45–52.

94. Wood, F.G. (2002) Ethnic differences in exercise among adults with diabetes. *West J. Nurs. Res.*, **24**, 502–515.

95. Umpierrez, G.E., Gonzalez, A., Umpierrez, D., and Pimentel, D. (2007) Diabetes mellitus in the Hispanic/Latino population: an increasing health care challenge in the United States. *Am. J. Med. Sci.*, **334**, 274–282.

96. Mokdad, A.H., Ford, E.S., Bowman, B.A. *et al.* (2000) Diabetes trends in the U.S.: 1990–1998. *Diabetes Care*, **23**, 1278–1283.

97. Cowie, C.C., Port, F.K., Wolfe, R.A. *et al.* (1989) Disparities in incidence of diabetic end-stage renal disease according to race and type of diabetes. *N. Engl. J. Med.*, **321**, 1074–1079.

98. Sands, M.L., Shetterly, S.M., Franklin, G.M., and Hamman, R.F. (1997) Incidence of distal symmetric (sensory) neuropathy in NIDDM. The San Luis Valley Diabetes Study. *Diabetes Care*, **20**, 322–329.

99. Resnick, H.E., Foster, G.L., Bardsley, J., and Ratner, R.E. (2006) Achievement of American Diabetes Association clinical practice recommendations among U.S. adults with diabetes, 1999–2002: the National Health and Nutrition Examination Survey. *Diabetes Care*, **29**, 531–537.

100. Perez-Escamilla, R. and Putnik, P. (2007) The role of acculturation in nutrition, lifestyle, and incidence of type 2 diabetes among Latinos. *J. Nutr.*, **137**, 860–870.
101. Thackeray, R., Merrill, R.M., and Neiger, B.L. (2004) Disparities in diabetes management practice between racial and ethnic groups in the United States. *Diabetes Educ.*, **30**, 665–675.
102. Poss, J.E., Jezewski, M.A., and Stuart, A.G. (2003) Home remedies for type 2 diabetes used by Mexican Americans in El Paso, Texas. *Clin. Nurs. Res.*, **12**, 304–323.
103. Hatcher, E. and Whittemore, R. (2007) Hispanic adults' beliefs about type 2 diabetes: clinical implications. *J. Am. Acad. Nurse Pract.*, **19**, 536–545.
104. Poss, J. and Jezewski, M.A. (2002) The role and meaning of susto in Mexican Americans' explanatory model of type 2 diabetes. *Med. Anthropol. Q.*, **16**, 360–377.
105. Packer, C.D. (2007) Type 2 diabetes and Hispanic culture: two kinds of insulin resistance. *South Med. J.*, **100**, 767–768.
106. Menselson, T., Rehkopf, D.H., and Kubzansky, L.D. (2008) Depression among Latinos in the United States: a meta-analytic review. *J. Consult. Clin. Psychol.*, **76**, 355–366.
107. Fisher, L., Chesla, C.A., Mullan, J.T. *et al.* (2001) Contributors to depression in Latino and European-American patients with type 2 diabetes. *Diabetes Care*, **24**, 1751–1757.
108. Young, A.S., Klap, R., Sherbourne, C.D., and Wells, K.B. (2001) The quality of care for depressive and anxiety disorders in the United States. *Arch. Gen. Psychiatry*, **58**, 55–61.
109. Lagomasino, I.T., Dwight-Johnson, M., Miranda, J. *et al.* (2005) Disparities in depression treatment for Latinos and site of care. *Psychiatr. Serv.*, **56**, 1517–1523.
110. Peek, M.E., Cargill, A., and Huang, E.S. (2007) Diabetes health disparities: a systematic review of health care interventions. *Med. Care Res. Rev.*, **64**, 101S–156S.
111. Wu, J.Y., Leung, W.Y, Chang, S. *et al.* (2006) Effectiveness of telephone counselling by a pharmacist in reducing mortality in patients receiving polypharmacy: randomised controlled trial. *BMJ*, **333**, 522.
112. Leung, W.Y., So, W.Y., Tong, P.C. *et al.* (2005) Effects of structured care by a pharmacist-diabetes specialist team in patients with type 2 diabetic nephropathy. *Am. J. Med.*, **118**, 1414.
113. Chan, J.C., So, W.Y., Yeung, C.Y. *et al.* (2009) Effects of structured versus usual care on renal endpoint in type 2 diabetes: the SURE study:

a randomized multicenter translational study. *Diabetes Care*, **32**, 977–982.

114. Fisher, E.B., Earp, J.A., Maman, S., and Zolotor, A. Cross-cultural and international adaptation of peer support for diabetes management. *Fam. Pract.* (in press).

115. Phillips, L.S., Hertzberg, V.S., Cook, C.B. *et al.* (2002) The Improving Primary Care of African Americans with Diabetes (IPCAAD) project: rationale and design. *Control. Clin. Trials*, **23**, 554–569.

116. Phillips, L.S., Ziemer, D.C., Doyle, J.P. *et al.* (2005) An endocrinologist-supported intervention aimed at providers improves diabetes management in a primary care site: improving primary care of African Americans with diabetes (IPCAAD) 7. *Diabetes Care*, **28**, 2352–2360.

117. Chan, J., So, W., Ko, G. *et al.* (2009) The Joint Asia Diabetes Evaluation (JADE) Program: a web-based program to translate evidence to clinical practice in type 2 diabetes. *Diabet. Med.*, **26**, 693–699.

118. Piette, J.D., Weinberger, M., and McPhee, S.J. (2000) The effect of automated calls with telephone nurse follow-up on patient-centered outcomes of diabetes care: a randomized, controlled trial. *Med. Care*, **38**, 218–230.

119. Piette, J.D., Weinberger, M., McPhee, S.J. *et al.* (2000) Do automated calls with nurse follow-up improve self-care and glycemic control among vulnerable patients with diabetes? *Am. J. Med.*, **108**, 20–27.

120. Fanning, E.L., Selwyn, B.J., Larme, A.C., and DeFronzo, R.A. (2004) Improving efficacy of diabetes management using treatment algorithms in a mainly Hispanic population. *Diabetes Care*, **27**, 1638–1646.

121. Rothman, R.L., Malone, R., Bryant, B. *et al.* (2005) A randomized trial of a primary care-based disease management program to improve cardiovascular risk factors and glycated hemoglobin levels in patients with diabetes. *Am. J. Med.*, **118**, 276–284.

122. Gollust, S.E. and Lantz, P.M. (2009) Communicating population health: Print news media coverage of type 2 diabetes. *Soc. Sci. Med.*, **69**, 1091–1098.

123. Cassano, P. and Fava, M. (2002) Depression and public health: an overview. *J. Psychosom. Res.*, **53**, 849–857.

124. Yeung, A., Neault, N., Sonawalla, S. *et al.* (2002) Screening for major depression in Asian-Americans: a comparison of the Beck and the Chinese Depression Inventory. *Acta Psychiatr. Scand.*, **105**, 252–257.

125. Chin, M.H., Walters, A.E., Cook, S.C. and Huang, E.S. (2007) Interventions to reduce racial and ethnic disparities in health care. *Med. Care Res. Rev.*, **64**, 7S–28S.
126. Dennis, C.L., Hodnett, E., Kenton, L., *et al.* (2009) Effect of peer support on prevention of postnatal depression among high risk women: multisite randomised controlled trial. *Br. Med. J.*, **338**, a3064.

# Acknowledgement

The World Psychiatric Association gratefully acknowledges the support of the following donors for this initiative: the Lugli Foundation in Rome, the Italian Society of Biological Psychiatry, Eli Lilly and Bristol-Myers Squibb.

# Index

Page numbers in *italics* indicate tables and figures.